Diabetes Type 2 and What to Do

Other books by June Biermann and Barbara Toohey:

The Peripatetic Diabetic

The Diabetes Question and Answer Book

The Diabetes Sports and Exercise Book
(with Claudia Graham, C.D.E., M.P.H., Ph.D.)

The Diabetic's Book: All Your Questions Answered

The Diabetic Woman (with Lois Jovanovic-Peterson, M.D.)

The Diabetic Man (with Peter A. Lodewick, M.D.)

The Diabetic's Total Health Book

Psyching Out Diabetes: A Positive Guide to Your Negative Emotions
(with Richard R. Rubin, Ph.D., C.D.E.)

Diabetes Type 2
and
What to Do

Revised Second Edition

by

Virginia Valentine, R.N., M.S., C.D.E.,
June Biermann, and Barbara Toohey

Foreword by Alan Marcus, M.D., F.A.C.P.

LOWELL HOUSE

LOS ANGELES

NTC/Contemporary Publishing Group

Library of Congress Cataloging-in-Publication Data
Diabetes type 2 and what to do / Virginia Valentine, June Biermann, and
Barbara Toohey.
p.   cm.
ISBN 1-56565-865-5 (2d ed.)
1. Non-insulin-dependent diabetes—Popular works. I. Biermann, June.
II. Toohey, Barbara. III. Title. IV. Title: Diabetes type 2 and what to do.
RC660.4.V35
616.4'62—dc20   92-37694

Published by Lowell House,
a division of NTC/Contemporary Publishing Group, Inc.
4255 West Touhy Avenue, Lincolnwood, Illinois 60646-1975 U.S.A.

Printed and bound in the United States of America
International Standard Book Number: 1-56565-865-5
10 9 8 7 6 5 4 3 2 1

I dedicate this book to my late mother,
Myrna Valentine, who was a Type 2 diabetic
and the epitome of what every nurse should be;
to my daughter, Melanie, who will most likely become
a Type 2 diabetic and who I hope will grow up
into a world without diabetes;
to the world's best husband,
John McLaughlin;
and to my adopted sister,
B. J. Christopher.
—V.V.

We dedicate this book to our good neighbors,
Lisa Granata and Linda Toth,
for their personal inspiration
and professional perspiration.
—J.B. & B.T.

CONTENTS

FOREWORD

The philosopher Peter Nivio Zarlenga said, "It is hard to begin to move when you don't know where you are moving, how to move, or if you are going to get there."

The path to your future good health begins with finding out that you have Type 2 diabetes. This is the moment of realization that your future is truly in your hands. At that moment, knowing you are diabetic, you are no longer the victim of an unseen enemy. You can begin to make decisions that will determine which path your life and health will take.

June Biermann, Barbara Toohey, and Virginia Valentine do not, to paraphrase Shakespeare, "rail against a sea of troubles, but indeed take arms against it and in so doing resist it." Type 2 diabetes mellitus, more than any other disease known to mankind, is "resistible." The patient with this disease is not doomed. Our knowledge as to the cause and nature of this disease has increased exponentially, and in Type 2 diabetes mellitus, knowledge is truly power. June, Barbara, and Virginia have given people with this infirmity the power to control their disease and influence their future. We have traveled a long path in a short time from the vision that things just happen at random to people with diabetes mellitus. Along the path, we have gained the understanding and the actions necessary to effect changes. As health-care professionals, we have learned that Type 2 diabetes mellitus demands to be taken as seriously as Type 1 and that the patient plays the most important part in the preservation of good health.

One cannot construct something of worth without quality tools and raw materials, just as one cannot embark on a path without a guide who is up-to-date, accurate, and above all, useful. The tools necessary to create the state we call good health are all presented by June and Barbara in their unique, straightforward, and always understandable and enjoyable style. What is found in this book will empower and serve as a road map to readers and enable them to take an active, enlightened, and vital role in the most important job they have ever had to assume to survive—helping themselves and helping others to guarantee the success of the treatment of a disease that above all else is treatable.

With this book we are not only given a road map, however, but also our own personal guide: Virginia Valentine. Like an experienced traveler who has been on a voyage of exploration, Virginia Valentine has come back home to help lead us all to the promised land. Rather than leading us at arm's length, as is all too often the way health professionals teach their patients, Virginia Valentine shares with us her own personal successes and failures, what caused them, and the results that ensued. She literally puts her arm around the reader and opens not only her mind but also her heart to her disciples and students, both new and old.

As one of the multitude who has watched the role of patients with Type 2 diabetes mellitus change from being the object of orders and the receptacle of instructions to the current and only acceptable role, that of equal partners in their health care, I am happy to be able to express from all of us to June Biermann, Barbara Toohey, and Virginia Valentine our heartfelt thanks for their book and their efforts, which have helped evoke this change in attitude and knowledge, and most important, for continuing to teach us and keep us on the right path.

Alan O. Marcus, M.D., F.A.C.P.
South Orange County Endocrinology
Mission Viejo, California

The Best Kind of Diabetes You Can Have

Several years ago a dermatologist removed a small growth near Barbara's left eye. The lab report came back indicating it had been malignant. The doctor was very reassuring. "It's all taken care of. You don't have to worry or even think about it. Just always wear a sunscreen when you're outdoors. It's the best kind of cancer you can have."

Many people who are diagnosed as having diabetes in their adult years are told something similar: "You have borderline diabetes," or "You have mild diabetes," or "You have a touch of diabetes; just stay away from sugar and lose some weight and you'll be fine." If the words, "It's the best kind of diabetes you can have" aren't actually spoken, the implication is there. And if it isn't there, you come up with it yourself. When June was diagnosed at age forty-five, she was disturbed and upset, of course, but kept saying to herself—and to anyone else who would listen—"At least I don't have the kind of diabetes that you have to take insulin for, so it's not so bad."

Later on when it turned out that she did have to take insulin after all, she immediately felt that her kind of diabetes was much more serious and that those who didn't have to take insulin really had it easy. She's ashamed to admit that once when she was feeling particularly frustrated and resentful over her own problems with diabetes, she bitterly referred to those who can get along on diet and exercise (or diet and exercise and pills) as "those fake diabetics." Her attitude was, "All they need to do is lose some weight. That's not hard to do." (This from a person who has been skinny all her life, has no taste for sweets, and isn't even all that much interested in food.)

But the more we learned about "the other diabetes" as author Doro Sims, who has diabetes herself, calls it, the more we learned that the grass is definitely not greener on one side of the diabetes fence or the other. Both sides have an equal share of weeds and bare spots, gopher holes, and snakes in the grass. We assure you that we're totally reformed now and we take all manifestations of diabetes equally seriously.

Unfortunately not everyone who has diabetes takes the condition so seriously. Whether their attitude has been fostered by reassuring doctors or self-created as a defense mechanism, the vast majority of people who develop diabetes as adults feel "it's not that big a deal" and go on to act accordingly: testing their blood sugars seldom or never, maybe exercising and maybe not, maybe changing their eating patterns and maybe not.

The more we saw this casual and lackadaisical approach to diabetes in action and the more we saw the health problems and diabetes complications that resulted from it, the more we realized that Something Had to Be Done. We wanted to alert this vast majority of diabetics to the fact that it is as important for them to handle their disease with serious care and attention as it is for those who have been shooting up insulin since childhood.

Because we have such great respect for diabetic endocrinologist Lois Jovanovic, M.D., with whom we collaborated on *The Diabetic Woman*, we wrote to her half-jokingly: "How would you like to put on 30 pounds and stop taking insulin? The reason we ask is that we really think there needs to be a book on adult diabetes. Janice, our editor, thinks so, too, because her mother just developed it and Janice is struggling trying to help her make the necessary changes in her life. We figured that if you wrote this book with us, it would give it that extra push of authority if you had Type 2 diabetes [the most typical kind for people diagnosed in their middle or later years]."

Dr. Jovanovic was quick to respond that she agreed such a book needed to be written, and that it would be a thousand times more meaningful if our collaborator had Type 2 diabetes. For that reason she suggested someone other than herself. Her recommendation was a person whom she described as "a Type 2 who uses her condition to motivate and win the hearts and minds of other Type 2s. She has won the 'Educator of the Year' award for the state of Oklahoma and the national award from the American Association of Diabetes Educators. She is witty, clever, and smart, too." She was referring to Virginia Valentine, R.N., C.D.E., formerly Clinical Nurse Specialist for diabetes at the University of New Mexico Medical Center in Albuquerque, New Mexico. She is also Clinical Associate faculty at the University of New Mexico College of Nursing.

Everything Dr. Jovanovic said about Virginia proved to be true—and then some!—as we quickly learned and as you will see in this book.

We will now put our three heads and two somewhat impaired pancreases together to help you develop an adult attitude toward your adult-onset diabetes, an attitude that will make it possible for you to make sure that your diabetes truly is the best kind of diabetes you can have—the well-controlled kind!

—*June Biermann and Barbara Toohey*

I Don't Have a Character Flaw— And Neither Do You!

I have had Type 2 diabetes for eighteen years. I was diagnosed at age thirty-one, which, as most textbooks will tell you, is much too young to get this type of diabetes. In the recent past, many times when I introduced myself to an audience, I would share with them the fact that I had Type 2 diabetes, but I always made sure to let them know that I was not yet forty. Too bad I can no longer use that disclaimer.

Most people, when they're diagnosed with diabetes, ask, "Why me, Lord?" But since there was so much history of diabetes on both sides of my family, I guess I always knew that eventually I would get it. My question was, "Why *now*, Lord? I wasn't supposed to get diabetes until after the age of forty. Although I felt a little cheated at getting it at such an early age, I wasn't all that worried because my paternal grandfather, who had diabetes, lived to be almost eighty, and my mother's diabetic aunts and cousins didn't have any of the terrible complications that I was to see later when I went to work in the field of diabetes.

I chose to go into nursing after several years in college as an art and advertising major when I realized that I wanted to do something that had a more significant impact on people. My mother was a nurse, but I had not previously considered nursing because I thought all nurses had to be as smart as she was—and I felt that let me out.

Then one summer after my sophomore year in college, I didn't have a summer job. Mothers can't stand it if they see you sleeping late and frittering away your time, so my mom made me come to the hospital to help out in the nursery. I was petrified of handling those little babies, but that summer I did discover two things that I'd not previously known or appreciated: (1) Most nurses were not as smart as my mom (which is not a put-down for nurses but praise for my mom, who was a genius), therefore I could probably handle the schooling; and (2) the essence of nursing is not shots and bedpans, but bringing out the inner healing reserves of people. That was the part of the job I really liked. I decided I would take college algebra and chemistry as a personal test to see if I could survive. I figured if I could live through those courses, I'd be able to manage nursing school. I could and I did.

In nursing school I discovered for myself something my mother had already told me: Medical patients are much more interesting than surgical patients. Medical service is where they put the older patients with chronic diseases. Among health professionals, the job of caring for patients with chronic diseases is not considered as glamorous as surgery, but I found the work much more rewarding and much more exciting. In medical service you get to know your patients and develop meaningful relationships with them.

A few years after graduating with a baccalaureate degree in nursing from Central State University in Oklahoma, I became pregnant with my first (and last!) baby. They told me I had gestational diabetes—that's the kind of diabetes that sometimes emerges during a pregnancy and then goes away after the baby is delivered. In 1976 most centers were not screening for gestational diabetes on a routine basis, but I was under the care of the university faculty, and they were checking for this. Although they recognized what it was, they didn't know much about treating it. Mainly what they did was to tell me to watch my sugar intake. (Sound familiar?) I followed their limited instructions except I didn't eat as many calories as they suggested. And still I had a 12-pound baby at full term. (In the past, overweight babies were typical for women with diabetes.) She was beautiful, 25 inches long, with thick, dark, curly hair. She made all the other babies in the nursery look anemic.

Then, just as the textbooks tell you, five years later I was diagnosed with diabetes. At the time I was in graduate school at the
University of Oklahoma College of Nursing specializing in chronic
disease, and my husband and I were in the process of getting a
divorce. (Could it be that I was under stress?) Since I was overweight
and had very high blood sugar levels, my doctor immediately put me
on insulin. I was on insulin for about a year before I decided to start
figuring things out for myself. I lost 50 pounds and got off insulin and
remained diet controlled for the next eight years. Nine years ago I
had to go onto oral hypoglycemic agents (pills) to control my blood
sugar, and weight control is a neverending battle for me.

In 1982, when I attended a diabetes management training program in New York with Dr. Lois Jovanovic, I learned that women
with diabetes didn't have to have 12-pound babies. To my sorrow, I
also learned that my child would be at a greatly increased risk for
Type 2 diabetes herself, not only because I had Type 2 diabetes, but
because she had developed increased fat cells during gestation. (I
think motherhood should be renamed guilthood.)

Melanie is now in her twenties and overweight. It's something
we have tried hard to avoid. We have watched the sugar and fat in
the house, but she has always had a big appetite, and year after year I
see her gain weight and struggle to deal with the excess weight and
the social problems it brings. I hope this book will be useful to her
when and if she does develop Type 2 diabetes and, before that, at the
time she is having children, when she will likely have gestational diabetes. (Fortunately, this is a long way off because I have told her she
can't have sex until she is thirty-eight years old.)

Since 1981 I've primarily worked in areas helping people with
diabetes. I love helping people with chronic diseases because they're
so downtrodden—the stepchildren of the health care system. It's
pretty amazing that people with diabetes are treated this way when
you think about it, since diabetes affects 6 to 10 percent of the population in America. I consider it a privilege to be able to make a difference for people who have my affliction. I am now a consultant for

health care agencies and the pharmaceutical industry, and I have a business in New Mexico called Diabetes Network, which provides diabetes education and case management statewide. I guess the reason I enjoy working with folks with diabetes so much is that I see the health care system and society in general treat them as if they don't have a real disease. Many people—and that includes many health professionals who should know better—treat Type 2 diabetes as if it is only the punishment for being fat. The implication is that if you weren't fat you wouldn't have the disease and, therefore, it's all your own fault. I know this is true, because I've had more than one physician tell me the same.

That's why my message in this book is this: *Diabetes is not a character flaw!* If you believe that you have diabetes because you're fat, ask yourself these questions: Why are there so many people out there fatter than you who don't have diabetes? Why do half the members of the Pima tribe of Native Americans in Arizona have Type 2 diabetes? Why do people with diabetes have parents and grandparents who also have diabetes?

I'll answer these questions for you. Type 2 diabetes in overweight people is a disorder in the way food is metabolized (converted to energy) and used in the body. Yes, lifestyle can affect diabetes, but when you look at the research reports on Type 2, you see that the origin is in the genes you're born with. It is genetically determined, just like the color of your eyes. (And nobody calls your blue or brown eyes a character flaw!)

Probably in the next ten years we'll see treatments directed toward the correction of these metabolic errors. What we have to do in the meantime is learn to live with the disease in such a way that we can stay healthy and participate fully in our lives. For me, participating fully in life means helping my patients and living in the mountains outside Albuquerque with the world's greatest husband and daughter. To do that I have to constantly work at diabetes management myself. The major challenge for me is to stay on a healthy diet and get some exercise every day.

The American Diabetes Association has as its mission "a world without diabetes." When I first saw that statement, I tried to picture a world without diabetes and I couldn't stretch my imagination to visualize such a thing. Maybe the end of Type 1 diabetes can be achieved, but I can't bring myself to even dream of a world without Type 2. I have to alter that phrase into "a world without *suffering* from diabetes." For me that means helping people keep their blood sugar in the near-normal range so they don't suffer the terrible, disabling complications of diabetes. It also means helping people make the necessary lifestyle changes for diabetes management without suffering—giving them commonsense approaches tailored to the individual. Above all, I want to keep them from feeling blamed for the disease they inherited.

For me, a world without suffering from diabetes is available right now, not something we have to wait for until a far-distant day. My reason for writing this book is to show you how, together, we can achieve this new kind of world for people with Type 2 diabetes.

—*Virginia Valentine, R.N., M.S., C.D.E.*

CHAPTER 1

TYPE 2 DIABETES:
The What, Who, and Why of It

June describes a scientific definition as "a term you don't understand explained in words you don't understand." Nowhere is this more true than in diabetes. When you're first diagnosed and have no idea of what diabetes is and how it's going to affect your life, *wham!*, you're hit with a whole bunch of scientific terms for your type of diabetes.

We don't want to start this book with a lot of confusing diabetilingo. On the contrary, our goal is to use what we might call "beginner's language" so you can gradually ease into a diabetes vocabulary that will serve you well over the years and allow you to communicate effectively with diabetes health care professionals (physicians, nurses, dietitians, etc.), allowing them to communicate effectively with you. Here goes your first vocabulary lesson.

First off, what is this thing called diabetes? It is a chronic (meaning it's for the rest of your life) physical problem that causes you to have too much sugar in your blood. Diabetes health care professionals often call the sugar in your blood *glucose*, a more specific (and scientific!) term. The medical term for high blood sugar is hyperglycemia (*hyper* in this case means too much, and *glycemia* refers to glucose in the blood). Low blood sugar is called hypoglycemia (*hypo* means too little). Euglycemia, a term used less often than the other two, means just right blood sugar—not too high and not too low—in other words, *normal* blood sugar, which is what nondiabetics have. The word *euglycemia* has the same prefix as euphoria—*eu*: a feeling of happiness and well-being. And euphoria is exactly what you'll feel when you get your hyperglycemia down to euglycemia. The goal of all the advice and counsel in this book is simply to move you into that ideal realm of normal blood sugar.

The American Diabetes Association defines diabetes as "a disease in which the body does not produce or respond to insulin (a hormone produced by the pancreas). Without insulin your body cannot properly convert the food you eat into energy." They go on to point out that diabetes is actually a general term for a number of separate but related disorders. "These disorders fall into two main categories: Type 1 and Type 2." And since you're reading this book, we're assuming you're a Type 2.

What is the difference between these two types of diabetes? That has recently been clarified in new guidelines announced in June 1997 (the old ones dated from 1979!) by an Expert Committee convened by the American Diabetes Association. Besides redefining the categories of diabetes, the Expert Committee converted the former Roman numerals into Arabic numerals to avoid confusion. (Virginia says she guesses they must have thought people would read the Roman numerals wrong and think they had Type 11, or eleven, diabetes.) All the older books of course still use Type I and Type II, but now you know better—and you'll know when you're reading an older book. You may still see in some books—and hear from some diabetes health care people—some of the now outmoded terms for Type 2, such as maturity-onset, non–insulin-dependent, or even NIDDM—non–insulin-dependent diabetes mellitus. (There's a term we won't miss!)

Here are the current ADA definitions of Type 1 and Type 2 diabetes (it pays to know the difference in case you haven't been correctly diagnosed):

In Type 1 diabetes your body destroys the cells in the pancreas that produce insulin, usually leading to a total failure to produce insulin. It typically starts in children or young adults who are slim, but it can start at any age. It afflicts about 700,000 Americans. In Type 2 diabetes the body cannot use insulin properly and sometimes doesn't produce enough insulin. It usually occurs in people over forty-five and overweight among other factors. About 7 to 7.5 million Americans have been diagnosed and another 8 million remain undiagnosed with Type 2 diabetes.

As we said before, in both types of diabetes the basic problem is that without treatment there is too much sugar in the blood. In this first chapter we'll ask Virginia to interpret and amplify these definitions and to explain how and why you became diabetic and in what direction you should go with your diabetes therapy to correct your abnormally high blood sugar.

—*June and Barbara*

DEFINITIONS OF DIABETES

JUNE AND BARBARA: Virginia, how do you explain to your patients what the meaning of Type 2 diabetes is and how they fit into the picture?

VIRGINIA: I think this new classification system is much clearer than the one we used to use. Of course, there are variations with the Type 1 and Type 2 groups. The variations could explain why most people get Type 1 diabetes before the age of twenty, and then some, like June, get it later in life. You can still tell the 1s from the 2s by the amount of insulin their bodies make. You can either do a C-peptide test (this indicates the amount of insulin being made by your pancreas) or you can use the less expensive alternative: Just take a look at their body shape. It takes insulin to store fat. By looking at me you can see that I make plenty of insulin. You can't get "fluffy" without insulin. June, on the other hand, has a hard time storing fat, and without insulin, she would rapidly drop weight. That's never happened to me.

Type 1s usually have an absolute insulin deficiency that could be caused either by an autoimmune process (the immune system gets confused and mistakenly destroys its own insulin-making cells) or by an idiopathic (of unknown cause) process.

Type 2 people, on the other hand, have what we call "insulin resistance." This means the basic problem starts with resistance to your own insulin at the muscle cell, so insulin doesn't move glucose into cells. Your glucose has no place to go so your blood sugar keeps getting higher. This alerts your pancreas to start making extra insulin to take care of the glucose. Eventually your insulin-making cells grow so weary of trying to produce enough insulin that they give up, leaving you with what we unscientifically—but accurately—call "pancreatic poop-out."

So if you have Type 2 you are considered "relatively insulin deficient." No, that doesn't mean your relatives are insulin deficient! It is important to realize that people with Type 2 are making insulin, but just not enough to overcome their resistance and keep their blood sugar normal.

JUNE AND BARBARA: How do you know the Type 2s are still making some insulin of their own?

VIRGINIA: We know because they rarely, if ever, go into diabetic coma, or, as we say in medical circles, diabetic ketoacidosis (often abbreviated DKA). DKA is caused by extremely high blood sugars from lack of insulin. The Type 2s are protected from DKA because they still make some insulin, at least enough so that some glucose can get into their cells and prevent the body from sending out the message that it's starving. That message tells the body to start breaking down fat and converting it to glucose. When this happens, the conversion of fat and protein to glucose leaves a waste product called ketones. These are acid products that are very bad for your body. When your acid base balance is upset, your normal metabolic processes cannot work. This is a serious medical crisis that calls for immediate hospitalization. Typically, Type 1 diabetics will report that especially at times of stress from illness they've had bouts of DKA. But it is unusual for an adult Type 2 to experience DKA, and if it does happen, it's usually at a time of extreme stress, such as a surgery.

JUNE AND BARBARA: That's certainly a piece of welcome news! Not only have the definitions of diabetes been revised but also the methods of diagnosis. What can you tell us about this?

VIRGINIA: Yes, the other big news from the new classification system is the blood sugar level number for diagnosing diabetes. If you have a fasting blood sugar (before breakfast) of over 126 mg/dl, you are now considered diabetic. (Note: Blood sugar numbers refer to milligrams [mg] of glucose per deciliter [dl] of blood. We often omit the mg/dl after the number in this book.) In the old diagnosis system, you weren't classified as diabetic until your fasting blood sugar was over 140 mg/dl. Many people already had the complications of diabetes (nerve, eye, and kidney damage) when their fasting level had reached 140.

The other problem with the old system was that you weren't considered diabetic until your blood sugar was over 200 two hours after a glucose challenge. It turns out when your post-glucose challenge glucose is 200, your fasting glucose is about 125. By diagnosing at or above 126, people can treat their blood glucose levels earlier and avoid many of the complications.

Another improvement is the recommendation for regular screening of the general population for diabetes. This is a real departure from previous standards. The U.S. Centers for Disease Control estimate that there are 16 million people with diabetes but one-third don't know they have it. (Funny how the CDC should know but the people who have it don't.) Because there are so many undiagnosed people out there, they now recommend screening all people over forty-five years of age every three years.

JUNE AND BARBARA: It's high time somebody woke up to the fact that much of the problem with the destructive consequences of undiagnosed diabetes can be prevented. June was diagnosed with a blood sugar of 425 (normal is about 70–120) and we're always hearing of those who only find out about their diabetes after their high sugars have given them significant symptoms of complications because they've already had the disease for many years.

Can you tell us how Type 2 diabetes slowly develops over the years and how it affects your body?

VIRGINIA: There are three problems that lead to Type 2. We'll take them in one-two-three order, although they don't necessarily develop in such a clear-cut way.

1. Insulin resistance and hyperinsulemia (too much insulin)

In Type 2 diabetes the insulin produced by your pancreas does not work as it should because over the years your body cells have become resistant to it. They don't accept it as they once did. (Scientists aren't sure yet why this happens.) The cells in your body have receptors which, if working properly, accept the insulin. This coupling triggers a chain of events that open the cells to accept glucose (the sugar your body uses as fuel). If muscle cells don't use the glucose, it will be stored as fat.

When your body notices that your insulin isn't working to move glucose into the cells, it gets busy and makes more insulin. You then develop what we call hyperinsulemia, or too much insulin in your blood. Insulin is a powerful fat-generating hormone. This extra insulin, then, causes you to store fat and to be very hungry. By eating more to satisfy your insulin-induced hunger, you add even more weight. The extra fat caused by too much insulin and too much eating further increases your insulin resistance. Putting the two together, you now have the initial insulin resistance caused by Type 2 diabetes plus the additional insulin resistance caused by being overweight—a vicious cycle if ever there was one!

2. Inadequate insulin production

Now we come to the second of the three problems that cause Type 2 diabetes. So far the story is that you started many, many years before with insulin resistance. This caused your body to make extra insulin to try to move the glucose into your cells so that your blood sugar would stay normal. You probably had a weight problem to begin with and gained more weight over the years because of the extra insulin. When, then, did you actually become diabetic? When your body could no longer make enough extra insulin to compensate for the resistance. Let me make it clear that you're not really deficient in insulin—you're making way over the normal amount—but what you make is not enough, considering your needs, to keep your blood sugar at the normal level, so you end up with high blood sugar. In other words, you have diabetes.

3. Excess liver metabolism

Now you're insulin-resistant, without enough insulin even though you're still making a whole bunch of it, and your blood sugar is higher in the morning than it was when you went to bed. The explanation for this is that you have developed what we call excess liver glucose production. That's right, just when you thought things couldn't get worse, your liver gets into the act. When you haven't eaten in quite a few hours (since supper), your liver thinks it needs to start giving back some of the glucose it has stored up for this kind of emergency. The liver either releases stored glucose or it can convert protein into glucose. When your liver starts kicking in after a six- or eight-hour fast, because your insulin resistance keeps the glucose from getting into the cells, the liver pours in extra glucose so you wake up with terribly high blood sugar, even though it was normal when you went to bed.

To sum up, you have a resistance to insulin so your cells can't make use of the insulin as they should. Your pancreas is making a lot of insulin but it's still not enough to overcome your resistance. And your liver doesn't understand why the glucose it's releasing isn't getting into your cells, so it does the only thing it knows how to do: It keeps producing more and more glucose, and that makes your blood sugar go higher and higher. That's how diabetes develops and keeps getting worse until you get proper treatment to bring it under control.

JUNE AND BARBARA: To help us better understand all this, could you tell us a typical story of how one individual's Type 2 diabetes might have developed over the years? Then each of our readers can visualize what probably happened to bring on his or her diabetes.

VIRGINIA: Yes, I can easily trace for you the physiological history of a typical case of Type 2 diabetes. Let's call the heroine of our story Helen. We'll say that she's fifty-five years old, overweight, feeling sluggish, has dry, itchy skin subject to frequent slow-healing infections, and has tingling in her toes. She makes a doctor's appointment, is examined and tested, and is diagnosed with Type 2 diabetes. (These are typical symptoms, but sometimes there are absolutely no signs that would cue the person to go to the doctor.)

Helen's Story

Let's go back ten to twenty years ago, when Helen develops the problem of insulin resistance (she is not aware of this, of course). To overcome this resistance her body starts making extra insulin to try to get the glucose from her food into the cells where it can be used as fuel. The extra insulin does keep her blood sugars normal, and therefore she is still nondiabetic. The extra insulin also causes her to gain weight, because it makes her store as fat a higher percentage of the food she eats. Soon she'll refer to herself as the type of person who can gain 5 pounds just smelling a plate of brownies—and she almost can!

After a few years, the excessive insulin she is making to compensate for her resistance is no longer enough. Now her pancreas starts losing its ability to produce the huge amounts of insulin she needs. My friend Dr. Lois Jovanovic calls this "pancreatic poop-out." Normally when a person starts eating a meal, the body sends out a little squirt of insulin within minutes. This is called the first-phase insulin response. You can control your blood sugar a lot better if you have insulin right there at the door to meet the food than if you have to conquer a high blood sugar after the meal. Helen's body now refuses to send out enough insulin to cover that first-phase insulin response.

Look at the diagrams in Figure 1.1. The first shows how the normal pancreas sends out a small amount of insulin at the beginning of a meal, followed by a second-phase response that sends out a larger amount of insulin to keep the blood sugar from going up after the finish of the meal. The second bump of insulin prevents blood sugar from going up more than 20 or 40 points (or mg/dl). (We use the term "points" for simplification. Thus, 20 points would be 20 mg/dl and 40 points would be 40 mg/dl.)In other words, the person without diabetes who starts out with a blood sugar before meals of 70 or 80 may go up after the meal to 110 or 120. It's not normal to have wide swings in blood sugars throughout the day.

The second diagram shows what happens to blood sugar levels when you lose the first-phase insulin response. The blood sugar spikes up way above normal levels until the second phase kicks in.

Figure 1.1 Insulin Response to a Meal

So without her first-phase insulin response, Helen is now beginning to cross over into diabetes territory. As her blood sugars climb, they tend to stay up. This is because it takes more insulin to conquer a high than to maintain a normal blood sugar. One year Helen's fasting blood sugar might be in the 90s and after meals in the 130s to 140s. A couple of Thanksgiving and Christmas celebrations later, she'll get fasting readings running 100–110 and get up to 150–160 after meals. It's something that just sneaks up on you little by little.

The phenomenon in which Helen's insulin doesn't work as well to conquer high sugars as it does to handle normal ones is called glucose toxicity. Blood sugar levels of 150–180 are considered toxic, because that's where the trouble that causes complications begins. These are the kinds of blood sugars that will lead to the fatigue, skin problems, and tinglings that will eventually cause Helen to go to the doctor.

Helen is now into full-blown diabetes but she doesn't know it. And that third problem we talked about before is setting in. Her insulin resistance is now so great that the cells in her liver that are supposed to notice all that insulin in her bloodstream have totally lost their ability to detect it. In the middle of the night after four or five hours of nothing to eat, her liver's job is to start putting glucose into her bloodstream as her blood sugar drops. The liver is a storage tank of fuel so that we never run out, even when we don't eat. Helen's liver, since it can't detect the presence of insulin in her bloodstream (its signal that there's food there), goes berserk. It pours out lots and lots of glucose. Helen gets excessive liver glucose production and delivery in the night, so she gets up in the morning with high blood sugar. That high morning blood sugar means she'll be high all day long, since her insulin no longer has the ability to bring down high blood sugars. When she finally goes to the doctor and has a blood sugar test, she'll find out why she doesn't feel well anymore.

"THRIFTY" GENES

JUNE AND BARBARA: Our next logical question for you is why do some over–forty-five and overweight people get diabetes while others go on blithely, getting even more and more overweight, but they never become diabetic. What factor(s) make the difference?

VIRGINIA: Type 2 is a genetic disease that runs in families. It is much more hereditary than Type 1. In studies of identical twins, in cases where one twin gets Type 1 diabetes, 40 to 50 percent of the identical siblings get the disease; when one twin gets Type 2, 90 percent of the identical siblings become diabetic.

JUNE AND BARBARA: In your introduction, Virginia, you mentioned that not only is there a Type 2 diabetes gene but also another genetic disorder that contributes to Type 2. We understand that this second disorder has to do with the way food is metabolized (converted to energy) and accounts for the way being overweight and getting diabetes go together (and they do go together because about 90 percent of Type 2s are overweight). Can you describe the metabolic error that causes the initial weight problem of most Type 2s, a problem that is later exacerbated by excess insulin production?

VIRGINIA: To understand this disorder we have to go back to our origins in this country—to the tribes of Native Americans who were here in the first place. I said that between 6 and 10 percent of the U.S. population has diabetes, but that's the overall figure. In Native Americans, Hispanics, and blacks the incidence of diabetes is more than 10 percent. Diabetes favors minorities, and the most favored of all are Native American citizens.

Native Americans are as much as 300 times more likely to get diabetes than Anglos. The professionals who work with the Indian Health Service explain this extraordinary rate of diabetes with the "thrifty gene" theory. This theory starts with the plight of the Indians a few thousand years ago. Imagine yourself living in America as a Zuni or a Sioux. You work from morning until night to get enough food to survive. Your food consists of fruits and berries gathered and perhaps corn grown in poor irrigation conditions. Your meat is lean wild game. Your life is one of strenuous hard work, and starvation is a major cause of death. Some persons evolve a metabolism that is very efficient and can "store" a higher percentage of food than other people. These are the people who will live through the winter, because they use less of their food for energy and store more of what they eat for times of famine. These are the ones who reproduce and pass on their life-saving metabolism.

JUNE AND BARBARA: That doesn't sound like a metabolic error, but more like a metabolic advantage.

VIRGINIA: Then was then and now is now. The advantage changes into a disadvantage when you take these people into the twentieth century. Give them cars and all the food they want, especially a diet high in fat (fat foods are stored as fat in the body more quickly than protein or carbohydrate foods), and you have people who gain weight very easily, coupled with a built-in genetic tendency toward Type 2 diabetes. These people have both insulin resistance and a metabolism designed to survive famine. With a body programmed like this, it's a real challenge to overcome civilization. After all, there have only been a few generations of Native Americans who have enjoyed ample food and modern transportation. And now we have to tell our Native American friends with diabetes to eat less and walk more. It's not surprising that many of them think we've lost our minds.

With this genetic double-whammy, the Indian people in America are being devastated by diabetes. In many tribes, as many as half the adults have Type 2 diabetes. Among Native Americans, gestational diabetes (a form that emerges during pregnancy) occurs in as many as 20 percent of pregnancies, compared to 3 percent in the rest of the population. This will only perpetuate the cycle. Amputations and kidney failure are occurring in the Native American population at rates that stagger the imagination. A couple of summers ago I visited the Hualapai tribe near the Grand Canyon in Arizona. This village of 1,500 people has a kidney failure rate 1,000 times greater than the national average.

Recently I was in Sacaton, Arizona, and had the opportunity to meet many of the Pima people, 50 percent of whom have diabetes. Let me tell you about Joy. She is thirty-six years old and has had diabetes for three years. It's not uncommon to find Pima children eight and ten years old with Type 2 diabetes. I talked with Joy about getting better control of her blood glucose levels without having to go on insulin. She's already at the maximum dose of oral hypoglycemics (blood sugar lowering pills). She was very receptive to trying a Fast Fast (carbohydrate-restricted diet; see Chapter 4) for a few days and then working on her diet, although I must tell you she was already doing most things right.

She told me she does not allow any cookies or chips in her house and wants to make sure her children eat right so that they don't get diabetes. That made me very sad, because it is not chips and cookies that are going to give her children diabetes. Of course, no one needs chips and cookies (except in rare emergencies), but we must not blame the disease on the patient. Joy will help her children eat better and live longer, because they're working on low-fat and high-fiber eating patterns.

For the sake of Joy's children and all the Pima children, I hope we will find the answer to prevent and cure this disease. All the Pima people I met are very concerned about their health and the well-being of their families. It's very disturbing to see the level of devastation that diabetes is causing in these lovely people.

WHO GETS DIABETES?

JUNE AND BARBARA: We're glad that the government has at last started a program to prevent Type 2 diabetes. The Diabetes Prevention Program for Type 2 is under way to identify people at high risk and to try different strategies to prevent insulin resistance. Some participants will receive counseling in diet and exercise and others will be given oral hypoglycemic pills or a placebo. Unfortunately, the results will not be available until 2002.

We know that besides the American Indians, the Hispanic population has a high incidence of Type 2—about 13 or 14 percent. Even more appalling, we've heard that 30 to 40 percent of Hispanic women over age fifty-five have diabetes. Why do Hispanic people also have such a high rate of Type 2 diabetes?

VIRGINIA: This is an interesting question, because if you go back to the Spanish ancestors of today's Hispanics, you do not find an increased rate of diabetes. The Spanish explorers who came to America brought a rich cultural heritage and horses, and some say they brought venereal disease, but it seems they did not bring diabetes to America. The Hispanic people of Mexico and the Southwest often forget that their Spanish ancestors who populated the area in the 1600s did not bring any women with them. Their high rate of diabetes is a genetic heirloom from the local Indian people with whom the Spanish mingled and married. People of Hispanic descent in America are ten to fifteen times more likely to develop diabetes than the Anglo population. Most of them will get Type 2 diabetes, although there are Hispanic people who have Type 1.

JUNE AND BARBARA: That brings us to America's black population. Ten percent of black Americans suffer from diabetes and it's the third leading cause of death in their racial group. An article in the February 1991 *Diabetes Forecast* explained that the high occurrence of obesity among blacks contributes greatly to this. And the main reason for their high rate of obesity (60 percent of black women over forty-five years of age are obese) is poverty and the diet that poverty imposes on them. Thirty-four percent of black men and women are below the poverty line, while only about 11 percent of white men and women are. Poverty and obesity, as the article puts it, often go together. Blacks also have "thrifty" genes because they're descended from Africans who had to hunt for food just like the early Native Americans did.

And now, Virginia, we finally come to people like you. You have those "thrifty" genes but you're an Anglo. Where do you fit in?

VIRGINIA: True, I'm not a Native American, even though I was raised in Oklahoma, nor am I Hispanic or black, but I got diabetes at a young age, just as some of the populations with high rates of diabetes do. In fact, they're getting it at younger and younger ages. I have a Norwegian grandmother and I have diabetes on both sides of my family. Lots of Northern European peoples developed the same "efficient" metabolism that allowed them to survive feast-and-famine lifestyles. In fact, Type 2 diabetes is increasing in the general population of the United States at the rate of 6 percent a year.

This brings me to something I heard the other day that goes along with this discussion of how Type 2 diabetes is Mother Nature's way of maintaining the species. An overweight Type 2 diabetic named Frank came into our center. Frank had been a prisoner of war in World War II, and when we explained to him how Type 2 diabetes works and why he has the problems he does, he got this sudden enlightened look on his face. "So that's why I never lost weight in the prison camp!" he exclaimed.

He went on to tell us how he had been in the camp for almost a year and was about the same weight when he came out as when he went in, while his comrades were reduced to skin and bones. He said, "Granted, I did get a little more food than my buddies did because I could speak Italian. I would go over and talk to the Italian prisoners and they would sometimes slip me a little pasta or something. But I certainly didn't get anywhere near the kind of food I needed, and yet I hardly lost any weight at all. I always wondered about that."

This is an excellent illustration of the fact that simply decreasing calories is not the way to lose weight. A low-calorie diet alone is absolutely not going to help the person with Type 2 diabetes. You see, the other aspect of being a prisoner of war was that Frank got almost no exercise, being confined to a small space.

What we're doing now with Frank is first working on having him cut down the amount of fat he's eating. But I've told him what I have to tell all Type 2 diabetics: His chances of getting down to an ideal body weight are two—a slim chance and no chance at all. So you see, it's especially important that we set other goals for ourselves: the goals of being healthy and fit. *Fit* means normal levels of blood sugar, normal blood lipids (the blood fats that can cause heart disease), normal blood pressure, and normal amounts of exercise in our lives. We should be able to walk and work and play and feel good. That's what's important.

HYPERTENSION AND DIABETES (SYNDROME X)

JUNE AND BARBARA: Since you've mentioned blood pressure, that gives us a chance to ask about another unpleasant statistic having to do with Type 2 diabetes. To us it's astounding that between 45 and 50 percent of Type 2s also have high blood pressure, and this is regardless of their ethnic background. How do you account for this and what does it mean?

VIRGINIA: It means that diabetes is more and more being recognized, not as a single disease, but as part of a group of diseases and possibly even the cause of all the diseases in the group. This larger problem is sometimes mysteriously called Syndrome X or, more descriptively, insulin resistance syndrome. I call it "hyperbetes," because its main features are hypertension and diabetes. Hypertension is the scientific word for high blood pressure.

I know this is a book about Type 2 diabetes, but we must look at the bigger picture. Over half the people with Type 2 either have or will get high blood pressure. The other diseases of Syndrome X are hyperlipidemia and atherosclerotic heart disease. Hyper-lipidemia means high levels of fats in the blood, and in this case more is not better. High levels of blood lipids and high blood pressure over time lead to atherosclerotic heart disease (ASHD). This means that the blood vessels serving the heart are getting clogged up; when one or more of them become totally clogged, it causes a heart attack. People with Type 2 diabetes die from heart disease more than from any other cause. When I am in the hospital to see patients, I end up spending more time on the heart floors than anywhere else, because over 30 percent of the patients there have diabetes. That is not a coincidence. This is why throughout this book we'll be talking about treating diabetes, but it may sound like we're treating heart disease instead.

JUNE AND BARBARA: We see there's a lot more to worry about than we realized and that we need to understand serious health problems other than diabetes. Why don't you take these terms—hypertension, hyperlipidemia, and atherosclerotic heart disease and define each of them for us before we go on?

VIRGINIA: Hypertension simply means high blood pressure. Normal blood pressure is about 120/80. Blood pressure over 140/90 is considered elevated. Hyperlipidemia means that you have high levels of lipids (fatty substances) in your blood. Blood lipids consist of triglycerides, cholesterol, and phospholipids. These circulate in your blood and are hooked up to proteins. That's why you may hear your doctor refer to them as lipoproteins. So now you may be asking, what are triglycerides and cholesterol?

Triglycerides: These are the main storage forms of lipids and constitute about 95 percent of the fatty tissue of the body.

Cholesterol: This is a natural component of cell membranes and is used to make other substances in the body, such as some hormones. Cholesterol can be absorbed from food or it can be manufactured by the liver. The kinds of cholesterol you hear about are HDL (high-density lipoprotein) and LDL (low-density lipoprotein). HDLs are known as "good lipids" because they are associated with decreased risk of heart disease. LDLs are known as "bad lipids" because a high level of LDLs has a strong and direct association with coronary artery disease. So you see, it is not enough to have a good total cholesterol anymore (under 200). You have to have high HDLs (above 50) and low LDLs (below 130).

Atherosclerotic heart disease: I've pretty much already described this one as fat-clogged blood vessels that can cause a heart attack. The problems that contribute to ASHD are diabetes, high blood lipids, high blood pressure, and smoking. Smoking more than doubles your risk of ASHD and it is something you can choose to do or not do. So don't do it!

JUNE AND BARBARA: Besides not smoking, what can you do about "hyperbetes"?

VIRGINIA: Hypertension and high blood lipids will improve if you follow our recommendation of a low-fat, low-salt diet and exercise. But remember that these problems are genetic and if they don't get better with lifestyle changes, there are excellent medications that will help. Check with your doctor regarding your goal range for lipids and have them checked at least twice a year. Have your blood pressure checked at least every three months and have a goal of a systolic number (that's the top number) of less than 130 and a diastolic number (that's the bottom one) as close to 80 as possible. This is referred to as 130 over 80.

   There are newer and better drugs for treating high blood pressure these days. They are classified as calcium channel blockers and ACE (angiotensin converting enzyme) inhibitors. They have been found to be especially beneficial for people with diabetes in that they may have a protective effect on the kidneys. Check with your doctor about whether these drugs would be suited for you. Also, blood pressure medication is like diabetes medication in the sense that you may need it for a while and then, with weight loss and exercise, you may be able to discontinue it. That's why it's important to see your doctor and get your blood pressure checked every three months so that he or she can adjust your dose as needed.

As you can see, "hyperbetes" is something we can all live with. One of our patients, Celia, is a good example. She came to us with all the classic symptoms. She had diabetes with a glycohemoglobin of 10+ (see page 30 for a definition), she was about 70 pounds overweight, and she had high blood pressure and elevated lipids. She had the hypertension part of the syndrome before the diabetes. At least, it was diagnosed first. She was put on a diuretic (water pill) for the high blood pressure and it did what diuretics often do—it raised her blood sugar. This is one of the reasons that diuretics are not the best drug group for treating high blood pressure in people with diabetes.

Celia was sent to us for diabetes education, and we realized that the diuretic was probably the culprit. We suggested she consult one of our endocrinologists. Our docs put her on a better regimen of blood-pressure-lowering medication plus oral agents for her diabetes. After a few months of working with our dietitians for diabetes control, she lost 22 pounds and was able to stop taking her blood-pressure medication, her lipid-lowering drugs, and her diabetes pills. So you see, the diabetes lifestyle—low-fat diet, weight loss, exercise—works to treat the "hyperbetes" syndrome. Celia was thrilled, and we'll continue to work with her to help her stay in good control.

Don't get me wrong. There is nothing wrong with medications for treating blood pressure, lipids, and diabetes. We would all prefer to get along without them, and often early in the disease that is possible. But when it is not possible, it's important to follow the prescribed treatment.

CHAPTER 2

WAYS AND MEANS OF CONTROL:

Doing What You Have to Do

Now we come to the major un-fun part of diabetes—the tedious part, the boring part, the relentless, day-after-day part. This is the testing of your blood sugar to see where you are and, in some cases, the taking of pills or insulin to get you where you want to be and keep you there.

Faced with this most unsatisfying aspect of diabetes, we need a little shot of philosophy. How about this one from Thomas Merton's *The Springs of Contemplation; A Retreat at the Abbey of Gethsemani:*

> If I insist that my work . . . mustn't be tedious or monotonous, I'm in trouble. . . . Time after time it fails to become so. So I get more agitated about it, I fight with people about it. I make more demands about it. It's ridiculous to demand that work always be pleasurable, because work is not necessarily pleasing. . . . If we're detached and simply pick up the job we have to do and go ahead and do it, it's usually fairly satisfying. Even jobs that are repugnant and dull or tedious tend to be quite satisfying, once we get right down to doing them. This happens when we just do what we have to do.

That's the way it is with doing what we sometimes refer to as "diabetic shenanigans." June tests her blood sugar six or seven times a day and takes five separate injections—sometimes more if she's sick or changing time zones or her blood sugars have gone haywire for some other reason. If she got agitated and fought with people about having to do this, she'd be a one-woman war zone. No, she just does what she has to do.

It's not likely that you'll have this much tedium and travail in your diabetic life, especially if you don't take insulin, but you still need to do what you have to do. And if you just do it without agitation, you'll find it's not so bad, maybe even quite satisfying, especially when you discover that you did what you had to do—and it worked!

There's another advantage to doing your diabetic shenanigans. It helps you keep your mind alert and your wits about you. Chief Justice Oliver Wendell Holmes, who lived to be ninety-four, kept his mind sharp right up to the end by doing crossword puzzles every day. Being diabetic means never having to look around for an activity to keep you on your mental toes. You've got one built in that will last your whole life.

So now Virginia will do what she has to do—show you what you have to do and how to do it so you can go forth and just do it!

—*June and Barbara*

GOALS FOR BLOOD SUGAR LEVELS

JUNE AND BARBARA: What do health professionals mean when they say a person with diabetes is "in control" or "out of control"?

VIRGINIA: This refers to how closely their blood sugars align with blood sugar goals. The general goals for diabetes control are 80–120 before meals, and 140 is the danger or "take action" level. What finally led to more realistic goals for control was the 1993 release of the results of the Diabetes Control and Complications Trial (DCCT). This ten-year study followed 1,441 people with Type I diabetes. It compared "conventional" treatment of two shots of insulin a day and one blood sugar test with "intensive" treatment of three or four shots of insulin a day and a minimum of four blood sugar tests a day. The DCCT proved that near normal blood glucose control can significantly help reduce the development of complications in Type 1 patients.

Well, we all knew that metabolic control really matters, but we had no idea how positive the study would be. It was better than we ever dreamed. Diabetic retinopathy was reduced by 76 percent, kidney disease was prevented or delayed by 56 percent, and neuropathy (nerve damage) by 60 percent. I went to the American Diabetes Association meeting in Las Vegas and sat in the front row to hear the news. I just knew that patients would be beating my door down when I got back to work. The response was underwhelming. Most patients still don't know, and most doctors still don't believe the results. Many doctors claim it only applied to Type 1 and didn't prove the effectiveness for Type 2.

Then, the Kumamoto study was published. This study replicated the DCCT on 110 Type 2 patients in Japan. Guess what? The results came out pretty much the same as the DCCT for eye and kidney disease and even showed a 50 percent reduction in cardiac events. All the Type 2s in the study were on insulin to manage their diabetes. Amazingly, there are still folks out there telling patients it's perfectly okay if their blood sugar is under 200. But now we know that good control makes a difference.

JUNE AND BARBARA: So what are your recommendations for each individual's goals for control now?

VIRGINIA: *Individual* is the correct word because goals should be established individually for each person. For instance, a person who is nearly eighty years of age doesn't need goals that aim for intensive control. This kind of tight control is ideally designed to prevent complications down the road. When you're eighty, the complications that you fear thirty years from the time of diagnosis are pretty insignificant. You can settle for blood sugars in a range where you feel good. No matter what your age, you deserve to feel good!

Again, in an elderly person severe hypoglycemia (low blood sugar) should be avoided because it can be dangerous. It could lead to a serious fall, for example. Depending on the individual, we might extend the goal range to somewhat higher than the tighter control levels generally recommended for younger people. We keep in mind, though, that if blood sugars go too high, the elderly person will not feel good and will be at increased risk of dehydration and infections.

The goals we would suggest for young people and children (not many Type 2s are in this age group) would be different. We might suggest the normal range of fasting blood sugars of 70–120 and one hour after meals of 100–160. We'd want to consider that this person has forty, fifty, or sixty years to live with this disease and we'd like to prevent complications.

For most Type 2 adults—neither the very young nor very old—we're happy with a before-breakfast blood sugar in the neighborhood of 80–120 and after-meal blood sugars of less than 180. Those are near-normal ranges, in other words, close enough to normal to prevent complications, yet not so close to normal that we're constantly battling hypoglycemia (low blood sugar) if the person is on medication.

Some Type 2s on insulin have severe hypoglycemic reactions with little or no warning. This sometimes happens to those who've had diabetes a long time. They lose their ability to sense the reactions. This is called hypoglycemic unawareness. Most diabetics can recognize an insulin reaction because of the typical symptoms of shaking, sweating, dizziness, poor coordination, and even less dramatic signs such as hunger, blurred vision, and irritability.

People who've developed hypoglycemic unawareness don't have these warning symptoms. They can get such a low blood sugar level that they suddenly pass out. This is why we tell them that it is their responsibility to test their blood sugar before they get behind the steering wheel of a car. Every time! And it should always be above 100 before they start out.

CHOOSING A DOCTOR

JUNE AND BARBARA: June was subject to hypoglycemic unawareness for many years. Her blood sugar could drop to 40 and she wouldn't even know it. The solution to this problem is to work hard to normalize your blood sugar and you will regain your symptoms of lows. June switched to the low-carbohydrate diet in 1995 and was able to stay within a range of 70–100. After about two months, she totally regained her hypoglycemic warning symptoms and can now tell at a level of only 60.

Let's switch now to another important problem when people are first diagnosed—and sometimes later on down the line. They ask, "How do I go about finding a physician who's really good at managing diabetes?"

VIRGINIA: My advice would be to ask other people with diabetes and get their recommendations. If you don't know any other diabetics (not likely these days!), you could call your local diabetes association and ask for the names of some doctors specializing in diabetes. If you don't have a local diabetes association, you could call a local hospital and ask which physicians on their staff specialize in diabetes. One thing to watch for when you're doctor-shopping is to find one who has a team of diabetes educators at his or her disposal. A doctor who does not use diabetes educator nurses and dietitians is not serious about managing diabetes.

JUNE AND BARBARA: Most people already have a family doctor, and so their question is likely to be, "Is it OK to stay with my family doctor to take care of my diabetes or do I need to go to an expert such as an endocrinologist or diabetologist?" Before you answer that, for the uninitiated, you'd better clarify exactly what these two specialists are and what they do.

VIRGINIA: An endocrinologist is an internal medicine physician who has had additional training in endocrine diseases (those involving the secretion of various hormones). Usually he has had an additional two-year fellowship and will probably be board certified in endocrinology. (Tip: Read the diplomas and certificates on the office wall.) Over half the patients of most endocrinologists have diabetes. It's by far the most common endocrine problem. Some endocrinologists refer to themselves as diabetologists because they specialize in the care of diabetes. A diabetologist can also be an internal medicine physician who did not take a fellowship in endocrinology but who specializes in diabetes in his practice.

JUNE AND BARBARA: Now that we know what endocrinologists and diabetologists are, let's go back to the basic question: "Do I need one?"

VIRGINIA: That's a question each individual has to decide for himself or herself. But there's help available in making your decision: the standards-of-care criteria written by the American Diabetes Association. These standards were developed by a consensus of top medical minds in diabetes and were designed to assure the best quality of care and also to be cost effective. They are available from your local ADA affiliate (call them and ask for reprint #CAIS335, which costs 45 cents). After reading them, you may ask yourself, "Am I getting this kind of monitoring of my progress and is my family physician capable of providing this level of monitoring?" If your answer is yes and you feel you have a good relationship with your doctor and are getting the continuity of care that is so important for a person with a chronic disease, then very likely you'll do fine with the doctor you have. It is also important, however, for you to have access to diabetes educators either through your doctor's office or elsewhere in the community.

On the other hand, an endocrinologist offers a different level of expertise in analyzing and treating the endocrine problems that you may be experiencing. You may need such help especially when you're just starting out your life as a diabetic. An initial consultation with an endocrinologist can get you off on the right track for the best level of care and diabetes control.

Many people will decide to stay with the endocrinologist either because they have difficulty in achieving control or because their care is complicated by another problem such as hypertension or a thyroid disorder, and they need the additional level of expertise of the endocrinologist in these areas.

Another time that an endocrinologist may be especially valuable is when you have had diabetes for many years and are starting to experience complications or are worried that you might develop them. In either case, you might need the services of an endocrinologist for complication screening and treatment.

JUNE AND BARBARA: Is it an either/or situation? Once you decide to work with an endocrinologist, must you say farewell to your family doctor and the longtime relationship you've built up with him or her?

VIRGINIA: Not at all. As I said before, you may feel you need an endocrinologist at the beginning and then, after you feel confident that your diabetes is in control and you can handle it, you can go back to your family doctor.

Then, too, you can be under the care of a primary-care physician and use an endocrinologist as a consultant who only works with you on your diabetes problems. Your family doctor is the one who takes care of your everyday sniffles and sore throats and flus and your other general medical problems. This is the best solution for many people.

JUNE AND BARBARA: Is the best solution always possible? Doesn't your health insurance provider or your HMO tell you what you have to do when it comes to seeking help for your diabetes?

VIRGINIA: That's true. Many times the third-party payment systems require that you go to your primary-care physician for basic care, and they only let you see an endocrinologist if your primary-care physician thinks it's necessary and gives you a referral to one.

JUNE AND BARBARA: What happens when you think you need to consult an endocrinologist and your primary-care physician thinks you don't?

VIRGINIA: Although that sounds like an impossible tug-of-war for you, there is someone available to put some weight on your end of the rope. Health maintenance organizations have care managers or benefit supervisors to help resolve such situations. They may negotiate with your primary-care physician to give you at least an initial referral or they may even assign you to a different primary-care physician. This latter might be the best idea, since if the disagreement has gone this far, it may have undermined the doctor-patient relationship to the point that you can no longer work effectively together.

Let me emphasize something here: It doesn't pay to be shy when it comes to your personal health care needs. Nobody is giving nice-guy points when it comes to taking care of your own health needs. You must realize too that no one—health professional or not—will take the level of responsibility for your health care that you yourself will. It is especially important for you to develop this attitude of self-responsibility in this day and age when all the health care systems are looking for the most cost-effective ways to deliver health care. You have to be strong, capable, and well-informed if you want the care you need and deserve.

JUNE AND BARBARA: That reminds us of our friend Jean, a college professor. She was in the hospital several days for extensive tests. Whenever she felt the care she received was inept or ineffective, she let the hospital staff know about it in no uncertain terms and demanded that the situation be rectified *immediately*. She almost always got what she wanted. As she was leaving the hospital, and had mellowed out somewhat because of the favorable results of her stay, she remarked to a nurse, "I guess I'm known around here as the scourge of the fifth floor."

"No," replied the nurse, smiling sweetly, "the scourge of the whole west wing."

Now, being obnoxious in general just because you're unhappy at being sick or incapacitated doesn't help matters in health care any more than it does in any other area of life. But we agree with Virginia (and know from our own experience) that a little scourging at the right time can work wonders when you are being denied the care—or the endocrinologist—that you know you need.

Before we leave the realm of the endocrinologist, is there any other time in life when a person with diabetes might require the services of one?

VIRGINIA: Absolutely! During pregnancy. Any woman with diabetes who is even thinking about having a baby should be under the care of an endocrinologist. In the first place, you want to be in good diabetes control *before* getting pregnant, since most of the damage the baby might receive from a mother with out-of-control diabetes takes place in the first trimester. Then, after you become pregnant, you'll probably also want to work with a perinatologist, a physician who specializes in high-risk obstetrics. If you can find a diabetes pregnancy team, this is the most effective way to manage the problems of diabetes and pregnancy. The "dream team" would consist of the following:

1. an endocrinologist
2. a perinatologist
3. an obstetrician
4. a diabetes nurse educator
5. a diabetes dietitian educator
6. a genetic counselor
7. a social worker

Call your local diabetes association to find such a diabetes and pregnancy program. It's certainly more complicated for a woman with diabetes to have a baby, but with the proper care and attention on her part and on the part of the health professionals she works with, she can have a healthy, happy baby just like any other woman.

GLYCOHEMOGLOBIN TEST

JUNE AND BARBARA: Lots of doctors don't seem all that interested in their patients' daily blood sugar tests. They act as if the only really important thing is the glycohemoglobin (hemoglobin A1c) test. Maybe you should explain what this laboratory test is and why doctors consider it so important.

VIRGINIA: I've known physicians who consider the glycohemoglobin to be the most important—if not the only important—test for their patients. To put it simply, this test analyzes how much glucose has bonded with your red blood cells and, thereby, indicates what your average blood sugars have been for the past eight to ten weeks (the time varies from individual to individual). It's a test that must be attended to since it most closely aligns with risks for the complications of diabetes. This makes it an extremely important indicator; a kind of shining beacon to the person with diabetes to illuminate what the future may hold. Certainly we all want to pay attention to the results of this test, to understand what it means, and, above all, to strive to stay within one to two points above the top of the normal range.

It's important for you to understand that in your glycohemoglobin test you don't necessarily have to get within the normal range for your particular lab value. That normal range is where people who don't have diabetes generally fall. If you're within the range that goes up to one to two points above normal, that is probably an acceptable level. For example, if the normal range in the test you're taking is 4–6 and your glycohemoglobin is 7, that's great, a good range. When you get close to 8, that's still OK, but not exquisite. Over 9, we're getting into the terrible range.

One problem with glycohemoglobin tests is that labs around the country vary in the numbers and in the process they use to do the tests. Consequently, numbers that are in the normal range in one lab's test may be abnormally high—or low—in another's.

JUNE AND BARBARA: That's certainly true. June recently took two glycohemoglobin tests. In one the "normal" range was 5.9 to 7.5 and in the other it was 3.6 to 6.0. We've recently heard about another type of test somewhat like the A1c. It's called a fructosamine test and you can do one yourself at home if you buy a special meter. How about that test?

VIRGINIA: I was given one of the new Duet meters at an educators' meeting and I tried a fructosamine or GlucoProtein test myself on the meter. Doing a test was as easy as doing a blood sugar test only it takes four minutes. The main advantage of the test is that it measures changes in control over the previous ten days to three weeks. I loved it because I could do it at home instead of driving somewhere to have blood drawn and waiting days for the result. Each test strip costs about $8. My fructosamine came out the equivalent of 6 percent on an A1c. This meter also tests blood sugar in only eight seconds. How would I use it? I think this will be a very useful piece of information for when you're changing therapy and a weekly or two-week average will let you know if it is working. Also, the test is very motivating. It's one more opportunity to take charge of your own control with an additional piece of information. The Duet meter is from the LXN Corporation of San Diego, California (1-888-596-8378).

Becton-Dickinson will be marketing a home A1c test that lets you put drops of blood on special paper and mail it in for the results. This will be at a cost of $20–$30.

If it's the glycohemoglobin or fructosamine test that's so important, why bother doing daily blood sugars? Because you can't fix a poor glycohemoglobin result unless you know what your daily blood sugars are—day in and day out—and work to improve those.

To sum up: The glycohemoglobin or fructosamine test is your long-term beacon. Your blood sugar tests tell you how you're doing in controlling your diabetes on a day-to-day basis. The daily tests give you the clues as to where your control problems are and what you need to do to improve. These two tests go hand in hand like love and marriage. Both are absolutely necessary if you want really good control.

URINE AND BLOOD SUGAR TESTING

JUNE AND BARBARA: Some people with diabetes are first told to test the amount of sugar in their urine in order to help with their control (this is the old-fashioned way), while others are put directly onto blood sugar testing. What is the difference between testing urine and blood?

VIRGINIA: It's very simple: Urine testing is worthless and blood testing is not. To go into a little more detail, urine glucose measurements are, as you put it, the old-fashioned way. Many years ago when there was no technology available for blood sugar testing at home, urine sugar measurements were thought to give some reflection of blood glucose variations that could be used to keep people in control. Since you don't "spill" (another old-fashioned term) glucose into your urine until your blood sugar is higher than about 180–200 (and even higher than that if you're older), then urine testing isn't going to be of much value. Added to that problem is the fact that urine glucose testing varies with the amount of liquid in the bladder. You may have had a spike of high sugar and then low sugar and you'll still spill glucose into your urine, even though at the time of testing your blood sugar is very low.

Let me give you an analogy. Testing urine for glucose control of diabetes is like driving a car using only the rearview mirror. As far as I'm concerned, it has no value. Some people say, "Yes, but it costs less money." Not really. When you consider the value of the information you get, it's extremely expensive. People also say that it's better than nothing. *Au contraire*. I'd like to assert that it's worse than nothing. Too often you're getting a false sense of security. Many Type 2 diabetics don't spill glucose into their urine until their blood sugars are in the 300 range (usually older people). As long as they're getting negative urine tests, they think they're doing OK, when in fact they're not.

Did I say urine test strips were worthless? Actually, they do have one useful function. They're great for testing "diet" soft drinks. Did you know that from 10 to 26 percent of fountain "diet" soft drinks may be regular soda instead? One of the teens we take care of did this test at a mall in Albuquerque. He used urine testing strips to test "diet Coke" ordered at all the places where it was available in the mall. More than 10 percent were the real thing and not diet. At one food outlet an employee confessed, "We were out of Diet Coke so we hooked up real Coke." Our patient explained to the employee that this deceptive practice could seriously hurt a person with diabetes. You can be sure the employee won't do that again.

JUNE AND BARBARA: We've had lots of people report this nondiet diet-drink phenomenon to us. Some who have checked it out have found even higher percentages of "mistakes," up to one-third the wrong thing. You can also use urine test strips to check salad dressings and sauces. If they register below 1/2 percent glucose on Tes-Tape or Diastix, they're probably safe.

Let's move on now to the subject of blood sugar testing, which is far from worthless.

VIRGINIA: Some patients do visual strip testing of blood samples. If money is an issue, then we have them cut their test strips in half with Chemstrips bg. Not only will it save money, but it's actually easier to read a half-strip against the color blocks on the bottle than it is to read a whole strip. On top of that it takes less blood. The way you do it is to cut the strip in half lengthwise. Just cut one at a time; don't do the whole bottle at once. And don't leave the lid off the bottle while you're cutting your strip—you don't want the rest of the strips in the bottle to deteriorate. This is a way to save a lot of money if you have to pay for the strips out of your own pocket.

JUNE AND BARBARA: Now we've slid gracefully into the next important question. Assuming cost is a prime consideration, at what time of day should people take their blood sugar tests and exactly how often? Different doctors suggest different schedules. Tell us what plan you recommend and why.

VIRGINIA: That depends on what information you need to know. Let me go through the different testing times and what they're telling you. First of all, most of you need to test your fasting blood sugar to find out how you're starting the day. This tells us how you're managing your blood sugar without the impact of food. Since most Type 2s have high fasting levels (remember that excess liver metabolism phenomenon), even though they may be better off the rest of the day, it's important to know that as well.

Now let's talk about testing after meals. If you really want to know how food is affecting your blood sugars, test an hour to an hour and a half after the meal. This is a true look at how the carbohydrate is affecting your blood sugar. For people using diet alone to manage their blood sugar, this is important information. Don't expect your post-meal blood sugar to be the same as your fasting blood sugar. Notice that when I gave you your goals for control there were two different sets, one for fasting and one for after meals. In our center, we like looking at the one-hour number instead of the one-and-a-half-hour number, because it more closely reflects how you're dealing with the food in that meal.

If you're on medication, that's a different story. Many times your doctor has instructed you to test before meals. This is the number you need to know to determine how well the medication is working. For instance, your fasting blood sugar tells you how well the oral hypoglycemic agent you took at supper is working or how well the long-acting insulin that you took last night is working. Many times if you get your fasting blood sugar in the normal range, then the rest of the day works out a lot better. Your before-lunch blood sugar is reflective of both the short-acting insulin that covered breakfast, as well as the long-acting insulin you take to cover the whole day. Sometimes you also have to look at your before-supper blood sugar to get an idea of how you might adjust your morning insulin. It also tells you how well the pill or long-acting insulin you took in the morning is working.

To sum it up for people on medication, probably a before-breakfast and a before-supper test plus an occasional after-meal test would be an adequate schedule. One of the after-meal tests could be done at bedtime. That gives you an idea of how supper is affecting your blood sugar and how well your blood sugar is in control before you go to sleep. If you take long-acting insulin and are very low before bedtime, you need to plan for a snack.

If you're the kind of person who does a lot of strenuous exercise (I hope you are), you should be testing right before your workout. If your blood sugar is below 150, have a snack before you begin your exercise. (The 150 may be a somewhat high or low number for you; it can vary with individuals and the intensity of the exercise.) For those of you on medication, this test is a useful tool to keep you at your best blood sugar level for exercise. Exercise lowers blood sugar. Many people also test after their workout.

You should definitely test if you're feeling the symptoms of low blood sugar (sweating, shaky, nervous, weak, confused). You need to see at what level your blood sugar causes you to have these symptoms of hypoglycemia. Some people get symptoms at 120, while others might not feel low even at 40. Anytime you feel hypoglycemic, test to see how low you are and if you really need to eat something.

JUNE AND BARBARA: So far we've only talked about visual test strips—those that you compare to a color chart. Easier to use and much more precise is the system where the strip is put in a meter that analyzes it and gives the result as a digital readout. There must be well over twenty models of blood-sugar-testing meters available now from different manufacturers, and new ones seem to be coming on the market every other day. They're all different prices and have many different features. Let's say you're a beginning diabetic, and your health insurance will reimburse you for a meter and the monthly supply of strips to use with it, or that you can afford to pay the expenses yourself. How do you go about acquiring a meter you'll be happy with and trust?

VIRGINIA: Let me give you a few criteria you can use:

1. Buy a meter made by a company you can trust. It doesn't neces-sarily have to be one of the major manufacturers that's been in busi-ness a long time. It could be a young company that's doing a good job of providing a meter system and support. But I'm always a little leery of a brand-new company with a brand-new meter. I can't tell you how many meters have come on the market for a short time, and then dis-appeared. Some models are shown at conventions for diabetes educa-tors and then never even make it to market. Many of my patients have been stuck with a meter from a company that doesn't support it. By support I mean the company has a tollfree phone number answered by knowledgeable, pleasant, patient customer representa-tives who are empowered to replace your machine quickly if you're having any problems. Also, they should provide easy-to-understand literature and instructions with the machine.

2. Buy a meter system that requires little or no operator technique. As far as I'm concerned, the easiest systems are those that do not require you to wipe the drop of blood off the test pad at a certain moment after you put it on. There are good systems out there—in fact, they're into second or third generation—that use wipeless strips. These advanced, leading-edge meters sometimes cost more than the old-fashioned meters. But don't be foolish and try to save 25 bucks up front on your purchase if it means you're going to be stuck with a sys-tem that requires careful technique and, therefore, has a lot of error built into it.

3. Go for a system that supports you in your lifestyle. If you're on the move a lot, go for a system that's small and easy to carry around, easy to use, with easily understood results, and that's accurate. If having a meter in your pocket or purse means you're more likely to do testing, then by all means, get an easily portable machine.

By and large, pharmacists are not experts on meter systems, although some have taken the time and effort to learn about meters. For the most part, pharmacists are experts on drugs and medications; they're not experts on the stuff in front of the counter. So I suggest you talk to a diabetes educator. The educator has training and experience with meters, has spent time out there with people who are actually using meters, and probably knows more about these systems than any other health professional, including your doctor.

JUNE AND BARBARA: Setting all those drops of blood to put on strips is no fun, as you well know. Many people—especially older people—have difficulty. Back when Barbara was teaching the use of meters and found someone who bled easily, she would go into raptures over them. ("You just bleed *wonderfully*! How lucky you are. If only everyone could get blood for their tests as easily as you do, this world would be a better place.") After you get the drop, putting it on the strip correctly can be an even greater ordeal. And when you botch the job, not only have you wasted an expensive strip, but you have to start all over again with a new drop. Do you have any magic solutions for avoiding all the above bloody mishaps?

VIRGINIA: I don't know if they're magic, but there certainly are solutions. If you're one of those people who don't bleed easily, you should wash your hands in warm water before taking the test. Next, hold your hand down at your side below your hips. If you're sitting in a chair, let your hand hang straight down for a few minutes. This will allow it to fill up with blood.

Some people who have a particularly hard time getting blood find they have to really milk the finger. In this case, it helps if you practice doing this motion the right way. Starting way down at the base of the finger near your hand, milk all the way down the length of the finger to the tip on the palm side of the finger until you get a big drop. Then let go of the finger. Let your finger pink up again, then repeat the milking motion. Some people make the mistake of constantly squeezing the finger, never letting go to allow the blood to come back into the finger.

You should always stick your finger on the sides instead of on the fingerprint surface. The "poochy" sides of your finger actually bleed better. Another thing I suggest is to always stick the underneath side of your finger as opposed to the top side. That way the blood goes onto the strip easily and correctly. If you stick the top side of your finger, the blood tends to drip into your fingernails. This not only makes it hard to get the right amount of blood on the strip, but it's unsightly to walk around with blood under your nails.

The typical textbook on diabetes tells you not to stick in the same place all the time because you will get a callus. Most experienced diabetics know that a callus can be rather welcome because finger pricks in a callus don't hurt. When you get a callus so thick that you can no longer get blood, then you need to move on to other areas.

JUNE AND BARBARA: The well-known diabetic diabetologist Peter Forsham also suggested using this callus technique if you're someone like a musician who's afraid of damaging your fingers with numerous finger-sticks. He advised a concert pianist to take the finger he used least in his playing and always take the test from the same place on that finger, causing a callus to develop there.

June figures that she takes over two thousand blood sugars a year but the punctures haven't ruined her fingers in any way. Is this an unusual experience? Do some diabetics have problems with soreness and damaged fingers?

VIRGINIA: Unfortunately, some people's fingers get so sore that they can hardly bear the thought of taking another blood sugar. That's why I personally like to stick only the three fingers that have developed calluses thick enough to prevent pain.

But it's also very important to find the right lancing device for you. Some stick way too deep for a particular individual. On the other hand, some don't stick deep enough to get the amount of blood you need for the test. Visit your diabetes educator, who usually has a whole drawer full of them. You can try out several to find the right one.

JUNE AND BARBARA: June likes the Auto-Lancet, which has a tip that adjusts with five settings to match your skin type. She's also found that the lancet can make a difference. Some brands of lancets may stick deeper or shallower and some brands are more painful than others.

VIRGINIA: That's certainly true. My favorite lancet of the moment is the B-D Ultrafine II. It has the universal fit for almost all lancing devices and is extremely fine and therefore virtually painless. In combination with the dial-a-depth lancing devices, you can really deliver the perfect drop painlessly. Boehringer-Mannheim has a new lancing device that lets you dial in the drop of blood, but you must buy their lancet to fit the lancing device. It's a very gentle system, but I personally don't like having different lancets for different lancers because patients get confused about what to buy and pharmacies are generally of no help with this kind of trivia. Actually, I use the lancets over and over so that a box really lasts me a long time.

JUNE AND BARBARA: What if you think the meter you're using just gave you a wrong result—a totally unexpected and inexplicable number? This phenomenon usually only happens with an excessively high result. (We all are usually quite willing to accept low readings as valid.) In the case of the "wrong" reading, the normal reaction is to start cursing the meter. Some people may even want to hurl the thing across the room. Some people may actually do it! What do you suggest doing in such cases?

VIRGINIA: This has certainly happened to all of us. Rather than cursing the meter and throwing it across the room, the first thing you would want to consider is whether this truly could be a meter error. As far as I'm aware, there hasn't been a meter made that won't give you an erroneous number at some point in its life.

To check this out, you should retest, but first you should do some troubleshooting. Check the meter to see if it's clean. Do a control test. A control test means using a drop of control solution that comes with your meter to see if the machine comes up with a number that falls within the acceptable range for the solution. The control test is good for checking both the meter and the strips. The problem is that it costs you a strip to do it.

If your meter has a "check strip," at this point it's a good idea to use one of those. Consider whether the temperature of the meter may be too hot or too cold, because that will affect how it is working. If, for example, the meter has been left in the car and is very warm or very cold to the touch, let it come back to room temperature before you retest. Then retest your blood, being careful that your technique is exactly right and that you're putting the right amount of blood on the strip and doing the timing correctly. This is why I prefer wipeless systems and systems that require very little technique. It's much easier *not* to make mistakes.

At this point, if the reading you get is drastically different from the first one, you have to ask yourself which reading was accurate. One way to do this is to test with a visual testing strip (Chemstrip bg, Glucostix). This visual test will give you a kind of ballpark reading and you can decide from that which of the drastically different readings is most likely to be the correct one and which was erroneous because of faulty technique.

If, however—as usually happens—both of your meter readings agree fairly closely, then you have to admit to yourself that your blood sugar is indeed in that range, surprising though it may be.

JUNE AND BARBARA: Let's talk about strips and meters and how the costs of both have changed. Back in the olden days when June first started testing her blood sugar, meters were expensive. Her first one, an Ames Eyetone Reflectance Meter, cost $350 *used*. Had she bought a new one, it would have been $650! On the other hand, at that time, strips were relatively inexpensive—45 to 50 cents apiece.

Then the meter manufacturers got onto the razor blade theory. That's the marketing idea Gillette discovered long ago. The razor is sold for very little because the manufacturer knows it then has a long-time customer for its blades, and the blade prices can be on the high side. As a result, meter prices have dropped to as low as $50; sometimes, if you trade in a meter from a rival company, meters are actually free. This is because the makers want you using *their* strips and not the competitors'.

Where is the best place to buy your meter?

VIRGINIA: I have found that if you're learning to monitor your blood sugar for the first time, you should purchase the supplies from someone who can provide individualized education on blood sugar testing in general and on the meter you're purchasing in particular. Some medical supply stores can do this, although sometimes you're getting your instruction from a clerk with no specialized training in patient education or monitors.

Overall, a diabetes educator will probably be your best resource for training, and many times the educator will provide you with a meter or direct you to the best place to get one. Then you can bring the meter in for your training during a visit with the diabetes educator.

It's true that the meter may be cheapest at a mail-order or discount pharmacy. If, however, because of lack of instruction, you do the test wrong and waste strips and get false readings that lead you to taking the wrong amount of medication, the savings wouldn't be worth it!

We've decided at the Diabetes Center that our main business is not selling meters, so we don't try to make a substantial profit on them. But because we include the cost of training from a certified diabetes educator in the price, you can usually get them cheaper at discount stores. We always suggest the discount or mail-order sources to our experienced patients who are upgrading to a newer model or who are buying a spare meter. You shouldn't have to pay for training if you don't need it. Still, it's a good idea to talk to your educator before you order some sensational deal from a catalog. We may be able to tell you why the meter is so cheap (for instance, it may be a meter that they're closing out because a newer and much better model will soon be available) or warn you of potential problems (such as you can only get the strips in Outer Mongolia on the fifth Tuesday of the month).

So my advice is to get your initial training from a diabetes educator and look for cheaper sources for subsequent meters.

JUNE AND BARBARA: One thing we've noticed is that people often don't want to pay for diabetes education. They're willing to buy equipment and supplies because those are things they can hold in their hands and carry out the door. But in reality, the most valuable commodity they can buy is a better understanding of diabetes care. There's a Chinese proverb that we particularly like: "Put your money in your head, and nobody can take it away from you."

Part of the problem may be that insurance companies are sometimes reluctant to pay for education. This is a penny-wise and pound-foolish approach, since well-educated diabetes patients are more likely to stay out of the hospital where they'll run up huge bills for the insurance company to cover.

VIRGINIA: I couldn't agree more! Many studies have shown clearly that patient education pays off in terms of reduced hospitalizations and better health outcomes for the person with diabetes. The news about reimbursement and insurance coverage for diabetes education and supplies is now mostly positive. In the last few years, twenty-four states have passed legislation mandating that health insurance companies pay for diabetes education and supplies. (New Mexico passed their bill last year.) In general, these statutes require coverage for diabetes education, meters, strips, and medications without regard to type of diabetes or treatment. Of course, states cannot make Medicare do anything, but Newt Gingrich and Bill Clinton actually agreed on something last year and signed into law Medicare changes that will make them pay for strips and meters for everybody, regardless of the type of diabetes or treatment. They will also start paying for diabetes education under Part B (the doctor's office payment). This will take effect in early 1999, and we don't know exactly how it will work and who it pays yet. Of course, all of us diabetes educators are hoping it requires the education to be done by an educator (CDE or RD) and not just pay the doctor for the usual ten-minute visit with no real diabetes education.

Medicare currently pays for diabetes education under Part A, which means it must be hospital based and outpatient. In New

Mexico (and in most of the other states with this legislation), it has really helped with getting insurance companies to cover diabetes education. My feeling is that most of the large insurance companies recognize the value of diabetes education in helping patients improve control, and they definitely appreciate the value of improved control. They needed education to be mandated so that it "levels the playing field." This means that all companies have to pay for the benefit and therefore the smaller companies don't have an advantage with pay-ing fewer benefits and therefore charging a lower premium. Speaking of the value to insurance companies, in December 1997, *Diabetes Care* published an article that demonstrated the impact of control on cost to health plans. This exciting information showed the increase in costs to the health plan of various HbA1c levels in patients who tested over 6 percent (see Fig. 2.1). This is an excellent resource to use when you're trying to get an insurance company to pay for some-thing to help you get into better control—it shows the value of con-trol to the payor!

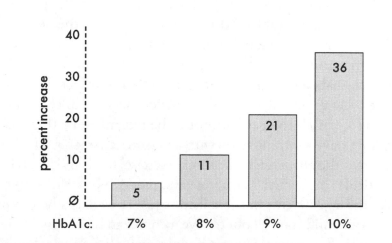

Figure 2.1 Cost to Health Plans of Poor Glycemic Control

Increase in medical charges over a three-year period for adults with diabetes and var-ious HbA1c values over 6%. Adapted from Gilmer, T.P., et al. "The cost to health plans of poor glycemic control." *Diabetes Care* 20(12):1847 (1997).

KEEPING RECORDS

JUNE AND BARBARA: Is keeping records of your blood sugar tests absolutely essential? Recording the results is a lot of trouble, and what good is it—especially if you keep getting more or less the same numbers and they're all too high? We've had people show us their records and have been amazed that day in and day out they'll write down the same 240s, 280s, or 310s and not question the pointlessness of keeping track of the same bad blood sugars without getting the message that *something different has to be done*. Surely blood sugar testing isn't an end in itself.

VIRGINIA: I agree that keeping records of blood sugars without taking any action is pointless. But I really encourage patients to keep track of their blood sugars while they are coming in for consultations with the diabetes educators. These records can help them identify areas of behavior that are causing them problems. For instance, we can correlate the high blood sugars with changes in diet, medication, or exercise. Also, by identifying patterns in the blood sugar readings we can help them change their medication to correct the problems.

But most importantly, while we're reviewing the records of their food intake, their blood sugars, and their exercise, we can help them learn our decision-making process. This is most important. Fine-tuning diabetes control is not rocket science. It's just being very sensitive to a person's lifestyle. We're never judgmental about blood sugars and we teach the patients not to be judgmental either. Blood sugars don't have anything to do with a person's character. They simply represent the effects of medication, exercise, food, and lifestyle on that particular individual. With time and practice you can learn how to make the adjustments in these factors just as well as a health professional can. And you will often have a choice in how to make these adjustments. For example, some people may choose to take more insulin or alter their medication to cover a particular meal or period of stress. Others may choose to exercise more. A lot of variations are possible. There isn't an absolute, rigid, you-must-live-this-way diabetes control program for anybody. We feel these choices should be left up to you, the patient. But you can't make these choices intelligently unless you're taught how. And you *can* be taught. Certainly if physicians can learn it and I can learn it and the health-care team I work with can learn it, you can learn it too.

We've learned it because we practice, but mostly we've learned it because our patients have taught us. We take our patients' records and examine them and have the patients tell us what happened. Then, when we've done this often enough, we come up with some guidelines.

For example, we may say, "Gee, it looks like every time somebody has had pan pizza, their blood sugars are much higher than when they eat thin-crust pizza. There must be a pattern here." You can do this kind of analysis on yourself. You can also see, using your blood sugar tests, the different effects of exercise and medication. It's really not a terribly difficult decision-making process. The important part of it is learning to be creative and flexible and to realize that there's more than one way to skin a cat.

MEDICATION: PILLS AND INSULIN

JUNE AND BARBARA: You mentioned in your introduction that you managed your diabetes with diet for eight years and now you're on oral hypoglycemic agents—or, as most of us call them, the pills. What are these pills, anyway?

VIRGINIA: These medications are specifically for the treatment of Type 2 diabetes. Now there are lots of new options compared to when I was diagnosed. We used to only have the sulfonylureas, which have been used for forty years. (This is pronounced sul-faw-nuhl-u-ree-us. It took me two years to learn how to say this. That's why most of us just call them "pills.") Now we have a wide choice of both the first-generation and second-generation pills. The second-generation pills kick your pancreas to make a little more insulin, making you more receptive to your own insulin at the cell receptor level. The second generation is more potent than the first and since they can be taken at a lower dosage, they have fewer side effects.

Among the new drugs that have appeared since 1995 are Glucophage (metformin), Rezulin (troglitazone), Precose (acarbose), and, in 1998, Prandin (repaglinide). Let me tell you about each of these and how it works and its drawbacks.

Glucophage (metformin) This is a recent cousin of a thirty-year-old drug. It can have some nasty side effects, but the trick is to not use it on people who are likely to get lactic acidosis (a side effect where the body doesn't eliminate wastes) as it can be fatal; some deaths have been reported from metformin. People who have kidney damage are also not candidates for this drug. Before considering the drug, you should have a creatinine level drawn. If it is above normal, your doctor may want to consider not using metformin. Another group of people at risk are those with poor liver function (people with abnormal liver function lab tests) and people who are binge drinkers or who drink significant amounts of alcohol. Additionally, people with congestive heart failure, COPD (chronic obstructive pulmonary disease), or any other serious disease should not be using metformin.

Now the good news. Metformin works by interfering with liver production of glucose. Since it works by a totally different mechanism than the sulfonylureas (they kick the pancreas to make it produce more insulin), it can be combined with them to work together. It turns out that either sulfonylurea or metformin will lower your fasting blood glucose about 50–60 mg/dl, but together they work better than either one alone. Most physicians still start with one of the sulfonylureas as the first-line therapy, but now many are starting with metformin and then adding the sulfonylurea for the second line. When starting metformin, it is important to begin with one tablet a day (500 mg) with a meal for a week or so, and then add another tablet with another meal. For example: Start with one 500 with supper; after one week add a 500 at breakfast and then add another 500 at supper. Most people need to get their dose up to 1,500 to see the effect. The maximum dosage is 2,500 but studies have shown that 2,000 is as effective as 2,500.

Precose If you are on the maximum dose of sulfonylurea plus met-formin, what do you do if your blood glucose levels are still elevated? The next step could be NPH insulin at bedtime or another one of the new available drugs. In 1996, a group of drugs called starch blockers came on the market. They block the effect of the enzyme that breaks down starch into glucose, so the starches are not absorbed at first. You know, eat a brownie . . . it goes away! Unfortunately, that is only part of the story. When you eat a brownie and have used one of these drugs with the first bite, it does not absorb in the first part of the small intestine. So imagine what starches do if they are not absorbed . . . they ferment. Then when they move farther down the intestine, they are absorbed. So you get all the calories plus gas!

The positive effect is that the post-prandial (after-meal) blood glucose is blunted. For a high-carbohydrate meal, you don't get such a high post-prandial glucose immediately after eating, and for some people, this improvement results in better blood glucose levels all around. In studies, the starch blockers resulted in about a 30 mg/dl reduction in fasting levels. The trade name of the blockers is Precose in the United States; other European versions may soon be available in the United States. One of the positive things about Precose is that it is not absorbed systemically, so it can be good for people who don't want to add another drug if they are already on a lot of different drugs.

Rezulin One of the interesting things about this drug is that the United States was the first to get it instead of the last, even though it came from Japan. Rezulin is the first pill that actually works at the cell receptor level. It stimulates muscle cells to make more of the transporter substance go to the cell wall and bring the glucose into the cell. We call this an insulin sensitizer. You may be asking, if this drug is working on the primary defect of Type 2 diabetes, why isn't it used as a first-line therapy? Studies show that Rezulin as a monotherapy only lowered the fasting glucose 38–48 mg/dl. The other problem is that it costs as much as $150 a month. Currently, it is most often used as an add-on after the sulfonylurea/metformin combination has pooped out. A patient can be taking as many as four medications plus insulin, so this is probably not the best way to manage diabetes and is certainly very expensive. The drug is relatively free from side effects except that a few deaths have occurred due to liver damage. Because of this rare side effect, liver function tests are recommended every month for the first six months and every two months for the next six months.

JUNE AND BARBARA: We used to think, the more pills the merrier, but you've shined a light on the situation that shows how complicated and even confusing the choices can be and how there's an unsettling period of experimentation involved for many people. We remember our former publisher, who has Type 2, was happy on metformin but tried Rezulin when it first came out. He found his blood sugars were much better on metformin so he switched back—and incidentally saved himself a lot of money. What has been your personal experience with all the new drugs and what combination have you settled on now?

VIRGINIA: Right now I'm on 20 mg Glucotrol XL and bedtime NPH insulin. This is a great regimen for me because I can do everything at bedtime. I take the Glucotrol XL and the insulin at the same time. The XL on Glucotrol means that it lasts twenty-four hours so it doesn't matter what time of day you take it. By taking NPH at bedtime, it helps turn off my liver so that my fasting glucose is much better. I take more or less NPH insulin depending on the amount of carbohydrate I had at supper and my bedtime glucose reading. I also take Humalog insulin for some meals and carry an insulin pen in my purse.

I've tried everything including metformin before it was on the market (I got it from Germany) and I couldn't tolerate it. It did help my blood sugars but I couldn't stay awake and I really felt bad. Last year I tried Rezulin and it is a wonderful drug. It cut my insulin requirement in half and improved my after-meal glucose, but, alas, I fell into the small percentage of people who are allergic. For me it caused significant swelling (my ankles looked like knees), which occurs in less that 5 percent of people. I haven't tried Prandin yet but I'm sure I will soon.

JUNE AND BARBARA: Should everyone who's having above normal blood sugars try the pills?

VIRGINIA: I know from my work with patients that there is no escaping the need for exercise and diet along with the pills or insulin or both. Insulin and pills are not a replacement for diet and exercise, they're just part of the armamentarium. Diet and exercise are still the key factors in managing Type 2 diabetes.

JUNE AND BARBARA: You mentioned that you now take insulin in combination with pills. Who decides that a person should go on insulin and how is this determined?

VIRGINIA: If you're on the maximum oral agent dose and your fasting blood sugar is still too high—and therefore your blood sugar will be too high for the rest of the day (as the fasting goes, so goes the rest of the day)—some physicians will add NPH (slow-acting) insulin at bedtime. By adding this dose of NPH, you can often normalize the fasting blood sugar. The pills will then work fine for the rest of the day. We call this BIDS: bedtime insulin, daytime sulfonylureas. It provides a nice alternative to having to go totally onto insulin. Also in selected individuals, we use the pills and insulin in combination to avoid going to much higher doses of insulin, which could predispose the person to weight gain.

JUNE AND BARBARA: Who makes the decision that a person should go on insulin and how is this determined?

VIRGINIA: Even though Type 2 diabetes is also called non-insulin-dependent diabetes, it's very common for Type 2s to go on insulin. This makes for a lot of confusion, because as many as 25 to 50 percent of Type 2s will eventually be using insulin to manage their diabetes. How is this determined? Typically, people with Type 2 diabetes, when diagnosed, can get along with diet and exercise. Then when their insulin production deficit becomes so large that they cannot overcome their resistance, they're given the oral agents. That works for a while. The average time that oral agents work is between five and seven years, although it can be much less time or even longer. I have a patient who has been on pills for twenty-five years. Granted, he's the only one I've seen who has made use of them that long. It's very unusual, but possible.

Now let's say that you've exhausted all efforts with diet and exercise and the oral agents are no longer controlling your blood sugar in the range that you and your physician have determined to be appropriate. Probably, your fasting blood sugars are significantly over 150 and after-meal blood sugars are significantly over 200. So you are told that you should go on insulin.

JUNE AND BARBARA: What happens next? How do you "go on insulin"? What kind of insulin and how much?

VIRGINIA: There are several different ways. Some physicians will simply take you off all oral agents and start you on an insulin regimen. Others in recent years have found that if they can just get the fasting blood sugar normal, then the rest of the day will be controlled just fine with pills. They may start you on one injection of NPH insulin at bedtime. NPH insulin is slow acting and has its peak action about eight hours after injection. The idea is that it will lower your blood sugar just about the time in the early morning hours that it ordinarily starts to go up because of excessive liver glucose production. This program, as I've mentioned, is called BIDS: bedtime insulin, daytime sulfonylureas.

If you fail on the pills, your physician may decide not to use pills at all anymore, but to go exclusively to insulin. Unit for unit, insulin is much cheaper than pills. If you're going to have to go on insulin anyway, some doctors reason, why not go straight to insulin to begin with and use insulin only? In that case, the 70/30 premixed insulin is ideal for Type 2 diabetics. This means that in any dose that you draw up, 70 percent of the units will be NPH-type insulin (slow acting) and 30 percent will be Regular insulin (fast acting). I favor this system myself, because it makes more sense for Type 2s. Remember, one of the three errors in metabolism that Type 2s have is abnormal insulin production. In other words, you don't get a first-phase insulin response. So when you eat a meal, you don't get that insulin right away to keep your blood sugar from soaring after the meal. That's why you need to have Regular (fast-acting) insulin or the new Humalog before breakfast, just like a Type 1 diabetic, and then NPH in the middle of the day to cover lunch. Notice, though, in Figure 2.2 that the NPH starts running out during dinner; that's the main reason most patients go on two shots a day of 70/30 insulin. This can be very convenient: just an injection before breakfast and before supper. It provides excellent coverage for most Type 2s.

On the 70/30 twice-a-day regime you'll need more insulin in the evening than in the morning. This is because your insulin resistance causes excessive liver glucose during the night. I tell my patients that we can't be shy about using as much insulin as it takes. The most important key for control in the Type 2 on insulin is to use as much insulin as it takes to get those blood sugars down. If you start out with a normal fasting blood sugar, it will take a lot less insulin to manage it throughout the day.

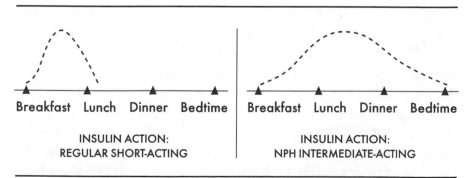

Figure 2.2 Timing of Insulin Action

Another common regimen uses NPH and Regular insulin that the patient mixes himself or herself. This is especially appropriate for Type 2s, because they do not have that cushion of insulin to keep their blood sugars relatively stable. NPH plus Regular is used before breakfast, Regular and NPH before supper, or Regular alone before supper and NPH at bedtime. Doing this allows you to adjust the Regular insulin doses based on your blood sugar level at the time and depending on what you plan to eat at breakfast and supper. This adds a certain level of flexibility.

Yet another variation is to use Regular insulin before each meal and not take any NPH until bedtime. This is the "treat only the problem" approach. Because some Type 2s have enough of their own insulin for basal coverage (baseline metabolism when not eating), they could have good blood glucose levels if they never ate (not a good long-term solution). If they take Regular before each meal and NPH before bed (some physicians prescribe Lente before bed), they're using insulin to supplement the problem areas during the day.

JUNE AND BARBARA: We notice that you've abandoned the old system of putting all Type 2s on just one shot of NPH every morning. That was certainly an easy way to go, and it was June's regime for years until she wised up and suggested to her doctor that she would like to use Regular before each meal. Is the one-shot-a-day system ever used today?

VIRGINIA: Yes, all too often Type 2s are put on only one shot a day. Almost always they should be taking more than one shot, and it should not be NPH alone. Let me explain why. NPH, as we noted, has a slow onset. It doesn't even start working for an hour or two, then it peaks in eight to ten hours and is usually gone in about fourteen hours. In other words, it doesn't last all twenty-four hours. If you take one shot of NPH in the morning, your blood sugar is going to go real high after breakfast, then a peak of NPH in the afternoon will pull you back down. That's not a good way to go. It lets the blood sugar fluctuate too widely during the day. It just doesn't feel good for our blood sugar to swing a hundred points. Mother Nature did not design us that way. We were designed to have a blood sugar fluctuation of no more than 30–40 points throughout the day. If we can mimic that for people with diabetes, they feel better.

JUNE AND BARBARA: There are so many kinds of insulin on the market now that a beginner might be very confused when trying to buy the particular one his or her doctor has prescribed. When June started using insulin twenty-five years ago, there were few choices, because we had only animal insulins (made from the pancreases of pigs or cattle). Now, of course, in addition to animal insulins we have the human insulins, which are exactly like the insulin the body makes. (Manufactured human insulin is made with recombinant DNA genetic engineering techniques.) Isn't it hard to explain all this to new insulin takers?

VIRGINIA: It's not really as complicated as it sounds at first. Only two companies in the United States make insulin: Eli Lilly and Novo Nordisk. And there are only five major types with different speeds of action.

1. Humalog is a new short-acting insulin, which is one of the great new inventions of diabetes care. It works like we always wished Regular (see #2) would work. It actually covers the meal! You can take it right before you eat and it acts within about 15 minutes. It peaks (has its strongest effect) in about 60 to 90 minutes and then goes away after about 2 to 4 hours. It has been shown to be quite effective for Type 2s who lack the "first phase" insulin production to cover a meal, even though they still make insulin.

2. Regular is the short-acting kind that starts working in about 45 minutes and peaks (has its strongest effect) in 2 or 3 hours and is gone in 4 or 5 hours.

3. The intermediate-acting insulins are NPH, by far the most commonly used, and Lente. (NPH stands for neutral protamine of

Hagedorn. Dr. Hagedorn of Denmark invented this insulin and named it after himself.) NPH starts to work in 30 to 90 minutes, peaks between 6 and 8 hours, and lasts about 12 hours.

4. The only long-acting insulin is Ultralente. The human kind has an onset of 1 to 3 hours, a peak that can span 8 to 14 hours, and lasts 18 to 24 hours. The Ultralente from animal sources has a delayed onset of 4 to 6 hours, a peak that can span 8 to 16 hours, and a duration of 25 to 36 hours.

5. There are several premixed combinations of NPH and Regular. There is the combination of 70 percent NPH and 30 percent Regular, which we favor in New Mexico for our Type 2s. And now a 50/50 mix is available. In Europe 60/40, 80/20, and 90/10 mixes are available. (Those Europeans must be pretty lazy if they don't ever want to be bothered mixing their own insulin dosage.)

6. In the near future, you will be able to get premixed combinations using insulin lispro (Humalog), as well.

As far as I'm concerned, cows should get beef insulin, pigs should get pork insulin, and people should get human insulin. I believe pharmacies could quit carrying all those formulations of animal insulin. I guess some people still take them just because they have never bothered to ask their doctor about switching. Why should you take human insulin? Because it's the insulin your body would make if it could. It is less likely to cause your body to make antibodies. When your body is making antibodies to the foreign protein in pork insulin or the three foreign proteins in beef insulin, then it is diminishing the effect of the insulin injection and possibly causing erratic action of that insulin.

Incidentally, there used to be another long-lasting insulin like Ultralente called PZI (protamine zinc insulin). It went off the market two years ago, but this didn't make the front pages of newspapers, because the only ones who missed it were cats with diabetes. It seems that veterinarians had found it to be the preferred insulin for diabetic cats. I'm sure vets have found a suitable alternative.

JUNE AND BARBARA: Doesn't taking insulin cause diabetics to gain weight? You've told us that it's a powerful fat-generating hormone.

VIRGINIA: Yes, it very well could. The person with Type 2 diabetes probably has enough insulin on board but is very resistant to it. Now we add more with injections. If you think about it, if your blood sugar has been running 250 and your weight has been staying stable, it figures that a fair amount of your calories have been going out in the toilet, because the extra sugar in the bloodstream is being spilled into the urine. If we give you enough insulin to get your blood sugar down to normal, those calories that were putting sugar into your urine have to go somewhere else, right? Probably right to your thighs.

    That's what I like about Humalog insulin. Since we don't have a first-phase insulin production to cover a meal, our blood glucose gets too high immediately after eating, which stimulates a really big load of insulin later . . . much later. All this extra insulin coming in several hours after eating only makes us hungrier and makes us gain weight. Humalog right before meals replaces our first-phase insulin response so that we don't have so much second-phase insulin and, therefore, have better blood glucose levels without so much hunger and weight gain. I'm using Humalog before meals when the meal has more than about 30 grams of carbohydrate. I think this is an ideal regimen for Type 2s who want flexibility of meal type and timing.

JUNE AND BARBARA: What's the best way to teach people how to inject insulin? Do you still use an orange to practice with?

VIRGINIA: Absolutely not! What a waste of a perfectly good orange. When a patient who has to go on insulin comes to me to learn how to inject, I don't talk about anything else, I just get straight to the injection procedure. I have them give themselves an injection using sterile water, so they can find out that it's not a big deal. It doesn't hurt if you do it right. Once they've done their first injection, then we can talk about other things such as managing their blood sugars.

    So many people have such an exaggerated fear of shots and

needles that we've had to come up with innovative ways to get them through that barrier. One thing I've discovered for people with severe needle phobia is never to use an alcohol swab to prepare for the injection. The smell of alcohol sends them back to being five years old and being chased around the doctor's office by a nurse who had to hold them down to give them a shot. So no alcohol swab. Just draw up the sterile water and inject immediately. Then they can relax because they know it's nothing. They've been worried so long, now at last they're relieved.

Using alcohol on your skin is really an unnecessary waste of money and cotton and alcohol. We tell people that the little germs on your skin have been buddies with your body for years, and nobody ever gets an infection from themselves. Lots of studies have been done on this. A study was even done of diabetic kids at camp. Can you imagine how dirty kids get? And none of them ever got an infection from their insulin shots. Another tip: You can reuse your insulin syringes. The label on a syringe says that you should use it once and then destroy it, but that's for hospitals, since needles are never shared between patients. When I recommend to patients that they reuse their syringes, they'll ask, "How many times?" My answer is that you'll know. When it bounces off your tummy, it's time to quit using that one. Most people find that after four or five times, they should switch to a new syringe.

BUYING SUPPLIES

JUNE AND BARBARA: We knew one man who always used his syringes around twenty-four times. He said he actually liked them better when they got dull! We also knew an environmentally concerned woman who searched in vain everywhere for one of those old glass syringes with detachable needles. She didn't want to load the landfill with disposable syringes. She finally had to compromise by using her syringes over and over again.

We consider disposable syringes to be one of the greatest improvements in diabetes injection ease. Are there newer ways to make insulin injecting, if not pleasant, at least more convenient?

VIRGINIA: Yes, there are many new ways to make your life much easier as far as insulin injections are concerned. A device called the insulin pen holds the insulin while you dial the dose. These pen devices are available in reusable models, which you load with a cartridge of insulin, or disposable models, which come preloaded and are disposed of when empty.

JUNE AND BARBARA: Some Type 2s may be interested in the insulin infusion pumps that are advertised as the best way to get good control. We know a lot of people who gained total happiness using a pump. What's your opinion of the pump system?

VIRGINIA: Pumps use what we call the basal-bolus insulin program. Basal refers to the insulin coverage needed to maintain blood glucose levels at times other than at meals. The bolus insulin (a concentrated dose) is used to cover meals. This schedule is designed to imitate the way your body handles its insulin output (a little bit all the time and more before meals). You don't have to be on a pump to use this system. You can use injections of Ultralente insulin morning and evening for a very nice basal effect and injections of Regular insulin before each meal. This gives you a lot more flexibility in being able to change your schedule, and being able to eat more or less at different meals. You can also exercise without having an insulin peak sneak up on you. We've had a lot of success with this program. Some people call it "the poor man's pump," because syringes cost a lot less than pumps.

The cost of pumps is the reason everybody on insulin doesn't use them. It costs around $5,000 to get started on a pump. For people who are very difficult to control, pumps are certainly a wonderful option, but most people who can manage their diabetes with exercise, oral agents, or injections see the pump as an unnecessary expense and more trouble to maintain than it's worth.

By way of example, I have one patient who is a Type 2 diabetic on a pump. She has had tremendous problems controlling her blood sugar for many years. She can take neither NPH nor Lente insulins because of allergies. She could tolerate Regular but didn't like taking injections five or six times a day. She finally came to me and said, "I want a pump." On the pump, her control was greatly improved. She enjoyed the ability to eat less at some times and more at other meals. She appreciated this new flexibility and ease of use.

She is a child psychologist, easily the best one I've ever met. When she got her pump and started it up, she noticed it made a clicking sound. With every little basal dose it gave, it clicked. She asked how to turn off the clicks. I told her she couldn't because that's how she knew the pump was working. She said, "The kids will go nuts over this. They're going to hate it and it's going to be distracting. This is going to be a big problem in my practice." She put the device inside an oven mitt and anything else she could find to muffle the sound. Then she started telling her young clients that she was a bionic woman and her body made clicks. They had no problem at all understanding that. It was only the parents who found her distracting. They were the ones glancing around the room with funny looks on their faces when they heard her click. By the way, she is now on a new pump, the Disetronic, that doesn't click, and she really loves it!

JUNE AND BARBARA: People who saw the movie *Reversal of Fortune* know that the contention of the prosecution was that Klaus von Bulow gave his wife a huge dose of insulin to kill her. She did not die but is in what appears to be an endless coma. Some moviegoers might have gotten the idea that insulin is a lethal drug or even a murder weapon. What are the real dangers, if any, of taking insulin and how do you set people's minds at ease on this score?

VIRGINIA: If you saw the movie, then you know what a bad idea it is to try to kill somebody with insulin. Granted that Sunny von Bulow is a vegetable today, but with normal doses of insulin the body has tremendous protective mechanisms to prevent problems from hypoglycemia. If your blood sugar starts getting too low, the pancreas starts increasing production of glucagon (the hormone that causes an increase in blood sugar; in other words, it has the opposite function of insulin). The glucagon tells the liver to start pouring out glucose.

Eventually the body will even start breaking down muscle and fat to make sure there is enough fuel available.

Under ordinary circumstances, even when a person's blood sugar drops so low that they pass out, which is rare and virtually nonexistent in Type 2s, the body uses counterregulatory hormones such as epinephrine to generate enough glucose to protect the body and especially the brain. These mechanisms provide enough glucose to revive you. With the massive doses of insulin that Sunny von Bulow received, her brain was allowed to go without fuel long enough to be damaged.

Unlike in Type 1 diabetes, Type 2s have such a huge level of stored glucose in the liver that they rarely experience any hypoglycemia, let alone pass out from low blood sugar. It is possible, though, to experience the feelings of hypoglycemia, even at a higher than normal level of blood glucose, if the brain has become what we call "glucose intoxicated." This means that if you are used to running blood sugars of 300 or 400 points and we quickly bring your blood sugar down to 150 or less, you may experience the symptoms of true hypoglycemia—for example, feeling shaky, sweaty, irritable, and headachy. This happens even though your blood sugar is at or near a normal level.

If this happens to you, eat a small snack such as a few crackers. Then with a little rest, the feeling will go away. We want to avoid overtreating that pseudohypoglycemia, because what will happen is that you'll just get your blood sugar back up to 300 and you'll never adapt to normal blood sugars. If you're used to running high blood sugars, you will usually adapt to normal ones in a couple of weeks. Then you'll feel better in the long run.

JUNE AND BARBARA: We've had many people come to us with the complaint that they suffer from hypoglycemia—the disease, not the hypoglycemic episodes that insulin-dependent diabetics sometimes experience. They're looking for books that might help them overcome the awful feelings of nervousness and depression that hypoglycemia causes. We don't know of any really good book for hypoglycemics, but we do warn them that we've heard this condition can be a precursor of diabetes. What we want to know is how is it possible to go from having a low blood sugar condition to the very reverse?

VIRGINIA: To understand that, all you have to do is remember that many, many years before being diagnosed with diabetes, the Type 2 diabetic lost the first-phase insulin response. If you don't have that first-phase insulin response, then when you eat a meal that is especially high in simple carbohydrates, you're going to get a real quick rise in blood glucose. This will stimulate an even bigger second-stage insulin response that in two to three hours will cause you to be hypoglycemic. We call this reactive hypoglycemia. This is the explanation of why many people tell you that they were "hypoglycemic" for years and then eventually turned into Type 2 diabetics, even though they seem like opposite conditions. Reactive hypoglycemia, in other words, can be one stage in the evolution of Type 2 diabetes.

I have patients who say that every time they eat a candy bar or drink a Coke they feel sick. There is a simple solution to this problem: Just don't do it! The diet for the person with reactive hypoglycemia is the same as for the person with diabetes. That is, eat foods high in fiber, low in sugar, low in fat—in other words, a good healthy diet. And don't ever drink liquid sugar—meaning soft drinks or fruit juice.

JUNE AND BARBARA: Is insulin a prescription drug in New Mexico? In California you don't need a prescription. How about other states?

VIRGINIA: Insulin is available without prescription everywhere in the United States. This is so it will be available in case of an emergency need by a person with diabetes. Some states, though, regulate the purchase of syringes and require a prescription for a syringe. Humalog currently requires a prescription but this will probably change in the next few years.

If you're going to be traveling, it's important that you carry your insulin with you and not check it with your luggage. But if you ever lose your insulin or run out of it, you can always get more. This is why it's important to carry a prescription or the name of your insulin so you'll know exactly what kind to buy. I always advise people who are first starting on insulin to tear off the box top and put it in their purse or billfold. That way they will know the brand name and type of insulin in case they're ever out of their home area and have to buy it.

Fortunately, in this country insulin is extremely inexpensive. This is rather surprising when you think about all the technology that goes into human insulin production using the DNA technique. Researchers have trained little bacteria or yeast to pump out the chains of amino acids that make up human insulin. (Come to think of it, though, they don't even pay these little workers minimum wage.) The insulin is as pure as it can get and it only costs $15 to $20 a bottle, which lasts most people three to four weeks. It is one of the cheapest prescriptions today.

JUNE AND BARBARA: If you want to do yourself in financially, just buy a bottle of insulin in Europe. In Switzerland it was going for $34 a bottle in 1992. And since foreign brands have different manufacturers and names for the various types of insulin, you can really get yourself in a bind if you leave home without enough extra bottles to see you through any emergency.

Unexpected things happen when you're out of your routine and in far-off places. June once left her insulin on the seat of the airplane when arriving in Hawaii. Fortunately, she called the airport and they held it for her even though she was silly enough not to have her name on the case in which she was carrying it. Another time her Regular insulin clouded up in France (the clouding was caused by silicon from repeated needle insertions into the bottle and was harmless, but she didn't know that). Then we had the experience of buying an insulin of a different strength (U40 instead of U100) and having to do complex calculations to get the correct dosage. Let her foolishness be a lesson to you (although most insulins are now the same strength abroad as here).

Since many diabetes supplies—insulin, pills, test strips—have expiration dates, how many weeks' or months' supply should a person buy? You don't want to run out, but you also don't want to let expen-sive products expire. There must be some way to be safe but not sorry when you look in your medicine chest.

VIRGINIA: When insulin is manufactured, a two-year expiration date is marked on the bottle. So the farthest out you can get insulin is a two-year expiration date, but one-year expiration from the time you purchase it should be more than adequate. You probably only need to keep a month's supply. Since the insulin you purchase from the drug-store has been carefully refrigerated, you'll want to keep your spare bottles in the refrigerator, too. (The insert in the Novo Nordisk insulins says, "Insulin should be stored in a cold place, preferably in a refrigerator.") The insulin you are currently using can be kept at room temperature and it can be kept for a month that way. If you're one of those people who don't use up a bottle in a month, I would suggest keeping it in the fridge and taking it out about an hour before you're going to use it. If you use it up in two or three weeks, leaving it at room temperature is no problem. (By the way, the inside of your car is not considered room temperature.)

Most syringes have an expiration date, but as long as they haven't been contaminated they're probably just fine.

JUNE AND BARBARA: What do you mean by contaminated? We've never heard of that.

VIRGINIA: Let's say you found them in the garage in storage and you see that years ago they got wet and have been chewed on by mice. Those syringes you'd want to dispose of. If they're still in their plastic bag or wrapper and have not had their protective covers removed and have not been through an atomic bomb attack, they should be OK.

JUNE AND BARBARA: So far June's syringes have survived a number of California earthquakes. But unlike syringes, pills can get out of date, can't they?

VIRGINIA: Yes, oral agents usually have an expiration date but that date is usually several years out, so that's no problem. The real problem with stocking up on any medication too far ahead is that if for some reason your physician should decide that you need to change the medication regimen, you're stuck with these drugs; you can't take them back. Could you use oral agents beyond the expiration date? Probably, but the pharmacists won't tell you that it's OK. I would talk to my doctor about this.

JUNE AND BARBARA: How about test strips? Sometimes people buy a lot of them at once to get a better price and then they find them going out of date.

VIRGINIA: Test strips are the one item to be careful with. They do go bad. I would watch the expiration date and I would not buy any strips whose date is not at least six months away. Granted, you would probably use them up before a slightly earlier expiration date, but it's best to be on the safe side. Strips are very fragile, and very sensitive to moisture or excessive heat. If left in the heat or the cold, in the car, or with the lid off the bottle—especially in the damp atmosphere of a bathroom—they can be damaged.

JUNE AND BARBARA: *Diabetes Forecast* publishes a "Buyers Guide to Diabetes Products" each year in its October issue. It's an extremely detailed listing and description of all products of all kinds, from carrying cases to insulin pumps to medical IDs. At the end is a complete list of manufacturers and suppliers with their addresses and 1-800 numbers. How helpful do you find this information, and what's the best way to use it?

VIRGINIA: The problem with this information is that there is no evaluation of the products. They list junk meters right up there equally with the quality meters. Therefore, there is no way to compare the products. Do I find this guide helpful? Not really. I already know the manufacturers' 1-800 numbers, but I guess for some people this may be a place to call and ask questions. I wish *Consumer Reports* would do an article giving a qualitative analysis of the different meters. Short of waiting for that to happen, you can always ask your diabetes educator. Your diabetes educator has probably had more experience with all of these products than any other single person and can help you decide on the best product for you.

JUNE AND BARBARA: Actually *Consumer Reports* finally did an evaluation of meters in their October 1996 issue. At the time, there were twenty-one different models on the market, but they tested only eight. They reported, "All meters we tested provided results that were accurate enough to be used with confidence." In their ratings, the Glucometer Elite (Bayer) and the One Touch (Lifescan) came out number one and number two.

What do you think of mail-order sources for purchasing supplies and equipment? About ten different ones in different states advertise each month in the "Shopper's Guide" section at the back of *Diabetes Forecast*. Others send out catalogs and newsletters. Have many of your patients used these services and found them advantageous?

VIRGINIA: Some people do like them, because they don't have to drive around town to find things. Having supplies delivered right to your door saves time. But often the prices of the mail-order supplies are very similar to the prices at the discount houses in your town, and buying locally saves you the cost of shipping, handling, and delivery (although if you're dealing with an out-of-state mail-order house, you can save the sales tax). I'd say it's a toss-up. Some people like mail-order sources and others don't find them to be advantageous.

CHAPTER 3

EXERCISE:
Your Lifetime Savings Plan

Personal finance expert Jane Bryant Quinn, in her book *Making the Most of Your Money*, advises that for lifetime financial security you should always "pay yourself first." By this she means that out of whatever dollars you make each month you should set aside 10 percent for saving before you do anything else with your money. Our advice for exercise is the same as hers for money. Before you plan anything else in your day, set aside 10 percent of your available time—for most of us that will average out at from thirty to ninety minutes—for exercise. Ms. Quinn is adamant that financial investment should be regular and inviolable; you should never say, "There's something I'd rather do with my money right now. I'll skip saving this month and double the amount next month." And we're adamant that exercise should be regular and inviolable; you should never say, "There's something I'd rather do with my time today. I'll skip my exercise and do twice as much tomorrow." The reason for both rules is that the saving and the exercise have to be a routine, a habit, and if you break the routine once it's easier to break it the next time . . . and the next . . . and the next, until you wake up one morning and find yourself in deep financial or physical trouble.

Ms. Quinn advocates different kinds of investments for different people. Some people aren't comfortable with the gyrations of the stock market and prefer mutual funds or the even more secure and stable money market accounts and T-bills. Some don't like the trouble of handling rental property, while others are willing to expend effort on property management in exchange for income and tax advantages. She even suggests a variety of investments for the same person to create a balanced savings portfolio and to avoid the risk of putting all your financial eggs in one basket.

We feel the same way about exercise. Some people like to play tennis, some enjoy square dancing, hiking, skating, walking, swimming, skiing, and, although most people don't or can't invest the time and effort it takes to run marathons, there are those who believe it's worth all the tremendous exertion in exchange for the mind and body benefits they derive from marathons. We also think that a balanced exercise portfolio is a good idea. Combining something that's aerobic with some strength training and possibly a competitive sport will give you activities to see you through all weather, seasonal, and personal mood fluctuations and will condition all parts of your body.

It's not easy to adhere to your savings program when you see others blowing their money on clothes or cars or vacations whenever they feel like it, with not a thought in the world for their economic futures. And it's not easy to stick to your exercise program when you're awash in a sea of workaholics who grind away fourteen hours a day and couch potatoes whose major exercise is reaching for a bowl of potato chips or punching buttons on the TV remote.

But the rewards are there for both Ms. Quinn's plan and ours. If you religiously follow her counsel, it's amazing the wealth you will be able to accumulate in a lifetime. You will be financially comfortable and secure when others about you are desperately floating loans or filing for bankruptcy or moving in with relatives. If you religiously follow our counsel, it's amazing the health you will be able to enjoy for your lifetime. You will be youthfully vigorous and vital when your contemporaries are sluggish and bloated and old before their time. On top of that, our plan has a big dividend, one that's as good in terms of your health as winning the lottery would be in terms of your wealth: *Your diabetes will be in good control.*

And here's the best part: Both these plans—the saving and the exercise—that are so beneficial for your well-being, can evolve into a joy and a pleasure if you enter into the spirit and make a challenging game of them.

We'll leave it up to Ms. Quinn and others to put you on the road to a lifetime money-saving program. We're here to put you on the road to a lifetime health-saving program and help you put your best foot forward.

—June and Barbara

BENEFITS OF EXERCISE

BARBARA AND JUNE: Virginia, you must be aware that both of us are exercise fanatics. We'll bet, though, that you didn't know we've written three entire books about sports—one on downhill skiing, one on cross-country skiing, and one on bicycling. And in 1977, with the help of 158 exercise enthusiasts who have diabetes, we published the first book ever to deal solely with exercise therapy for diabetes: *The Diabetic's Sports and Exercise Book; How to Play Your Way to Better Health.* Then, in 1995 we did an update of the book, changing the title to the more politically correct *Diabetes Sports and Exercise Book.* We were happy to collaborate with Claudia Graham, who has a Ph.D. in Exercise Science, a master's degree in Public Health, and is as Certified Diabetes Educator. But, her best credentials are that she has diabetes and is a near fanatic (like us!) when it comes to exercise. We learned a lot from her, much of which we'll pass on to you here.

Another thing we learned was how our diabetic exercise enthusiasts had fared over the last eighteen years. Of course we couldn't track them all down. Many had moved and many of the women had changed their names. Even so, we found enough to make us more convinced than ever that sports and exercise have ongoing, health-producing benefits for people with diabetes. And it's not just physical health. From the upbeat, positive attitudes they exhibited in their responses, it was easy to see that their mental health was in as great shape as their bodies.

We still feel just as passionately about the value of exercise for people with diabetes as we did then. And more than ever we keep preaching that others should become as fanatic about exercise as we are. Now that we've revealed our prejudice up front, we'll ask you how you rank exercise as a part of diabetes treatment.

VIRGINIA: Probably when the whole truth is known, it will turn out that exercise is everything. But, frankly, it's the hardest thing for me to get a grip on. I know that when we find the gene for Type 2 diabetes, he will be stretched out on his back with his feet up! I've not met one Type 2 who *loves* to exercise. It's a constant battle for us to get out and hoof it down the road even though it's the most important part of keeping diabetes in control.

Once again, I go back to the idea of living like our ancestors: being very physically active and eating a low-fat, high-fiber diet. The diet is much easier for me to master than the exercise. I constantly battle with myself to get out there and get moving. When other people talk about how good exercise feels, I wonder if there's some genetic reason that we Type 2s don't get addicted to it. Is it related to the fact that we don't use glucose the same way "normal" people do?

JUNE AND BARBARA: We can see, Virginia, that you're dragging your feet on exercise even while recognizing and acknowledging its crucial importance. So why don't we trade places in this chapter? We'll try to be so convincing about exercise that you'll find yourself skipping out the door with breathless anticipation.

VIRGINIA: I jump at the chance to accept your offer. Or, considering my feelings about exercise, maybe I'll just go stretch out on my back with my feet up and listen to your every word. Go ahead, convert me.

JUNE AND BARBARA: First, we want to make a little philosophical statement. We think every nurse and doctor—and every person with diabetes—should cease calling exercise a prescription, as in the question, "What is your exercise prescription?" or "This is your exercise prescription for the first month." Don't ever think of exercise as a prescription—some kind of bitter pill to swallow for your own good. Think of it as an opportunity to have fun, to go out and play the way you did as a kid.

Now, having put you in the right frame of mind, we can show you what exercise can do for you and how to get yourself doing it.

VIRGINIA: All right, what *can* exercise do for me? (I'm afraid I already know the answer to this!)

JUNE AND BARBARA: We know you know all the merits of exercise for people with diabetes, but in a sense you don't. As one of Leo Buscaglia's wisest teachers said to him: "To know and not to do is not to know." Maybe it's like taking skiing or tennis lessons. You hear the same thing over and over from different instructors until one day something clicks and you finally really get it. So here we go.

Exercise makes everything about diabetes therapy easier. It makes it easier to:

- control your blood sugar
- lose weight
- keep fit in the cardiovascular sense
- lower your blood fats
- increase your muscle strength and flexibility
- deter the "inevitable" process of aging
- avoid complications
- keep your spirits high and enhance your appearance and self-esteem

VIRGINIA: As a health professional, I concur with your entire list. I might add that the most important thing exercise does for overweight Type 2s is to change their metabolism so that they burn more calories even if they're sitting still. The books that explain this phenomenon best are those by Covert Bailey, who first published his *Fit or Fat?* in 1977, and since then *The New Fit or Fat?* as well as *Fit-or-Fat Target Diet*, *Fit-or-Fat Recipes*, and *Fit-or-Fat Woman*. What he says, over and over again, is that "the ultimate cure for obesity is exercise."

JUNE AND BARBARA: Yes, we've been preaching the Covert Bailey gospel since he came out with his first book. What people loved about his program was that initially he recommended a total of only twelve minutes of continuous aerobic exercise three times a week. That's not much time to give up for so much in return. Have you had any patients who have used the Covert Bailey program and found it helped them lose weight and significantly improve their diabetes control?

VIRGINIA: Yes. Lois is a patient who has the enviable life of spending half the year in Albuquerque and the other half on a lake in Michigan. (You get to guess which half where.) She has done an incredible job of managing her diabetes with exercise and diet. My partner, LaVerne, first started working with Lois while she was on insulin. With daily exercise Lois was able to lose 50 pounds and now has perfect blood sugars with no medications. She enjoys hosting students in her home who come to Michigan for music camp, including my daughter, Melanie, who says, "Lois is rad."

So it's agreed, exercise makes all our diabetes goals easier to achieve, but how can you make exercise itself easier? That's my problem. Although I love Covert Bailey, he hasn't been able to seduce me yet.

SETTING GOALS

JUNE AND BARBARA: You just start exercising. To begin, take whatever baby steps you have to—even if you exercise only four or five minutes a day. *Thinking* about exercising is what's hard. If you start doing something—almost anything—you're on your way. You've probably heard the saying, "Appetite comes with eating." Well, motivation to exercise comes with exercising.

Of course, there are some strategies and tricks you can use to get you going and keep you at it. The first strategy is to block out a time slot. Any time is great, though some experts especially recommend walking after meals. Back when we were working long hours in the SugarFree Center, the only way we could get in our exercise on weekdays was to do it right after breakfast. June did one half hour on a Schwinn Aerodyne (which provides both arm and leg exercise) and Barbara did a half hour of aerobics on a trampoline. On the weekends we would bike or walk. Now that we aren't tied down to an 8:00 A.M. to 5:00 or 6:00 P.M. schedule (we can just work all the time, weekends and holidays included), we try to walk 3 to 4 miles after breakfast three or four days a week. Initially, we went to a gym for upper body strengthening at least twice a week. But as the gym grew increasingly crowded (they kept offering membership specials), we grew increasingly impatient at waiting for the equipment, bailed out, and started working out with hand weights at home for our upper-body workout. If you do happen to join a gym and want to avoid the crowds as much as possible, we suggest going at 1:00 P.M., after the lunch crowd leaves. The best time of all is early Sunday morning since most of the workout-crazed yuppies are sleeping in after their big Saturday nights.

What we're trying to emphasize here is that you should work out your time schedule to fit your own life and sports activities. Everyone can do it! If you have to cut down on your time reading the newspaper or chatting on the telephone or playing bridge or watching TV, that's what you have to do.

Actually, cutting down on TV-watching is one of the best things you can do for yourself. A New York Times article told of a study by psychologist Robert Klesges of Memphis State University. He discovered that when children watch television, "they lapse into a deeply relaxed, almost semiconscious state . . . between resting and sleeping." This lowers their metabolic rate so that these children burn fewer calories watching TV than they would if they sat still doing nothing and almost as few as if they were sleeping.

Dr. Klesges believes that this TV-induced drop in metabolic rate could be a major contributor to obesity. In other words, it's the opposite of Covert Bailey's exercise-induced revving up of the metabolism. So cut down on TV-watching. It will prevent softening of the body as well as softening of the brain.

But whatever other activity you have to give up, just don't chicken out with that tired old excuse, "I have no time for exercise."

VIRGINIA: You're getting awfully serious about this. OK, I'll find a way to make the time. But I confess that I'm still reluctant. You said it was easy to get yourself in motion.

JUNE AND BARBARA: Maybe you're reluctant because you have no specific goals. Nothing is accomplished if you don't figure out beforehand exactly what it is that you want to accomplish. So here's our pitch on goals.

Set short-term goals by the week

Your goal must be specific, concrete, and realistically ambitious. (You can read about the art of setting goals in our book *Psyching Out Diabetes*, written with Dr. Richard Rubin.) A main point to remember is that the goal must be one you really want to reach. It won't work to let your spouse or even your doctor set your goal. If you set it, you're much more likely to accomplish it. It's OK to let your friends and family know your goal, as they may be able to help you stick with it.

Don't set your goals too high

This is another of the basic rules of goal setting. If you're thinking of jogging, for instance, you begin with half-mile runs, and then eventually you might want to work up to something as grandiose as 5 miles per week and in a few years 20 miles per week. All the new books on exercise emphasize that you should start out slow; the more out-of-shape you are, the slower you should start out. In fact, we've heard that to get in shape, it takes a month for every year you've been out of shape. For some of us that adds up to quite a chunk of time.

Have a goal of do-it-every-day

For people with diabetes, it is preferable to have the goal of exercising every day rather than the usual three or four times a week idea that has been so prominent in health advice. This is because it's easier to balance your medication and adjust your diet with daily activity. (There are exceptions, which we will explain.) One excellent walking program, *Walking Off Weight*, by Robert Sweetgall, Roba Whiteley, and Robert Neeves, advocates an eight-days-a-week goal, and that means walking not only every day but sometimes twice in one day so that if you miss a day occasionally, you'll still have done seven workouts a week.

Covert Bailey, who several years ago was preaching his twelve minutes of aerobic exercise three times a week as a total program, has switched to new advice: "Exercise longer, not harder." He has learned that his original method of having people use the formula 220 minus their age to get their maximum heart rate to set their exercise target zone is not effective for about 30 percent of the population and was causing a lot of people to overdo or underdo. (Approximately 15 percent of people have a slower heartbeat than the average and 15 percent have a faster heartbeat.) Now he emphasizes that "exercising at low levels is far, far more beneficial than we originally thought." One of his new rules is to "exercise as much as possible." And he's recommending that even beginners exercise six times a week for twelve minutes.

We might sum up by saying that your goal should be to try to get some exercise every day, even if it's only a few minutes and even if it's done in more than one short session. (See how reasonable we are?) As cardiologist James Rippe, director of the University of Massachusetts Medical School Exercise Physiology Lab, says, "You don't have to turn your life upside down to do things that have a profound impact on how happy, productive, and healthy you are." He recommends a simple two-step plan to feel better and reduce risk of heart disease: (1) Eat cereal with skim milk for breakfast, then (2) go out for a fifteen-minute walk. This simple plan works just as well for people with diabetes.

VIRGINIA: What a relief to know that I don't have to aim for exercise workouts that leave me sweating and panting and exhausted. I'm getting a little more enthusiastic. Do you have any more motivators in your gym bag?

JUNE AND BARBARA: We always have more! To impress yourself with your spectacular progress in fulfilling your goals, keep records, or as the sportspeople call it, a logbook. These records can be as simple as jotting down the day of the week, the time of day, the kind of exercise, and the length of time you exercised. You can use an ordinary monthly calendar with large squares for each day. Or if you keep blood sugar and medication records in one of the logbooks provided by meter companies, add your exercise record to this.

At the end of each week, total your time and see if you achieved your goal or how close you came to it. Maybe you even surpassed your goal and you can crow about it.

VIRGINIA: That's easy enough. When do we get to the hard part?

JUNE AND BARBARA: There really isn't any hard part—except maybe in certain people's minds. What we're coming to now is the *easiest* part—the reward or celebration for achieving your goal. We ourselves have gotten this down to a science. We have a reward not every week, month, or year but *every day*. This is the way it works. It's two miles from our house to the Coffee Roaster on famous Ventura Boulevard in the San Fernando Valley (just over the hill from the more famous Hollywood Boulevard). The Coffee Roaster is the neighborhood vendor of freshly roasted choice gourmet coffee beans, featuring outstanding cups of coffee, cappuccinos, and espressos and featuring owner Dick Healy's own fresh, home-baked fruit muffins (low in sugar and moderate in size). June takes her blood sugar—it's usually low after the two-mile walk—and then she's eligible for the reward: coffee and a blueberry, cherry walnut, or peach muffin, or whatever is in season. The muffin—or sometimes half of one—is just enough fuel to sustain a return trip.

So all you do is find a spot that's far enough away, a spot with something good to drink and/or eat, and take off. If you don't live in an area as coffeehouse filled as ours or don't like coffee or tea, you can carry your reward in your backpack and sit and enjoy it at the midpoint of your walk. This is just one idea. There are many nonfood rewards—even such schemes as putting 10 cents in a piggy bank for every mile or minute you walk. This is also a good way of keeping track of how long you exercise each day. The money saved this way is, of course, a discretionary fund to spend in any wild and crazy and impractical way you choose.

There are probably some saintly people out there who don't even crave such material rewards. Their reward is the inner satisfaction of achieving their goal and feeling healthier and more energetic, looking better, and enjoying life more.

STRETCHING

VIRGINIA: You're right about the importance of goals. Almost all successful people work with goals and rewards. I'm sitting here wondering, though, about the next problem that has popped into my mind. What kind of exercise are Type 2s going to do?

JUNE AND BARBARA: No matter when, where, or what kind of exercise you're doing, you should always begin with stretching. This increases flexibility and helps prevent injuries in whatever activity you follow it up with. Barbara even found stretching had curative powers. To "celebrate" June's twenty-fifth diabetes anniversary, we did what is known as *Wanderjahr*. When German students finish college they often take a year off for travel. We didn't take a year off, but we traveled a lot: Hong Kong, Bali, Wyoming, Paris, Florence,

Switzerland, plus a number of local trips. Wherever we went, Barbara carried a heavy bag full of cosmetics and diabetes supplies, including food for emergency situations, on her shoulders. When the year was over, Barbara's back was so stiff and painful from being thrown out of alignment by that bag she could hardly swing her legs out of bed in the morning. On her orthopedist's advice she started a program of stretching exercises. She also put a bowl of rice and chalk under her bed beneath the area where the pain was greatest. This was something she'd read in a book about Chinese medicine. In a few months the pain went away, never to return. (She still stretches every morning and the chalk and rice remain under her bed.)

Claudia Graham provides some good stretching tips in *The Diabetes Sports and Exercise Book*. For almost all stretches it's best to stretch slowly to the limit of regular joint motion. Stop when you feel resistance, before you feel any pain. Hold the stretch for about twenty seconds, because when the muscle is first stretched, the nerve impulses signal the muscle to contract (it thinks it's being overstretched). When you hold for twenty seconds, those nerve impulses go away, the muscle relaxes, and you have a greater and less painful stretch.

People are not rubber bands. Too-aggressive stretching (rapid bouncing and twisting) can cause injury. Always perform a more progressive, non-ballistic stretch. Cold muscles resist stretching, so some warm-up activity is a good idea. Always stretch before vigorous exercise, as well as afterward to prevent sore muscles. It makes a lot of sense to stretch daily and to incorporate stretches into your regular exercise program.

A few words of caution: If you're out of shape, have limited hip flexibility, or have a history of back problems, check with your doctor first. If you have proliferative retinopathy you may need to modify some of these stretches. Once you have gotten the go-ahead from your doctor, remember these tips:

1. Pay close attention to technique.
2. Never bend from your waist by rounding your back.
3. Bend at the hips and knees while keeping your back straight.

4. Don't hold your breath while bending, because that can cause a rise in pressure. (It's best to exhale as you stretch.)
5. Proceed slowly and hold for about twenty to thirty seconds. If it hurts at all, let up on the stretch.
6. Do a warm-up activity before stretching. (Even a hot shower will help.)

You need to stretch different muscle groups depending upon your exercise activity. But this is only an introduction to "Stretching 101," so we recommend an excellent book by Bob Anderson, called *Stretching*, with examples for every sport. (See Recommended Reading).

At first, stretch four times with a rest between repetitions. Try to do each stretch at least three to four times a week. It may take you a while, but by initiating your stretches for a few seconds eventually you'll be able to hold a stretch for twenty seconds.

VIRGINIA: It appears that stretching exercises are themselves a mini-workout. I like the cat's way better—one nice stretch upon waking. But I do see the logic of Claudia's stretching exercises, and warmed-up muscles are necessary for launching into the more strenuous activity that we always recommended at the Presbyterian Diabetes Center—aerobic exercise that benefits people with diabetes in particular. By aerobic I mean an activity that is continuous and rhythmic and done at a level that feels somewhat difficult. This means walking, jogging, running, bicycling, rowing, swimming, jumping rope, aerobic dancing, roller skating, and treadmill walking.

JUNE AND BARBARA: Aerobic is the word, all right. And you've given us the main choices, except maybe cross-country skiing, which is the most intensive workout of all. Your selection of sport is controlled to some extent by where you're going to be exercising: at home, in your neighborhood, or in a fitness center or gym. The aerobic possibilities in each of these locations differ.

In your home

If you can't leave the house because of weather, small children, hazardous neighborhood, or physical problems, then your exercise will depend largely on in-house equipment. You buy what you like and what you can afford. We've mentioned trampolines and jumping ropes, both inexpensive but quite intensive. More pricey (in order of least expensive to most expensive) are rowing machines, cross-country skiing machines, exercycles, treadmills, and stair-climbing machines. A good treadmill can set you back a pretty penny, say, $1,200 to $3,000. The popular stair climbers or step machines cost up to $5,000. (June's orthopedist warns against the stair-climbers because they're too hard on the knees.)

In judging equipment, you have to be certain that you aren't going for something that will stress your back or your bad elbow or whatever other physical injuries or debilities you may have. There's a lot to think about, so be wary of fast-talking salespeople who are themselves athletic types and don't understand that all of us are not as young and/or in as prime physical condition as they are.

Last there is the gentlest, least-damaging exercise of them all, swimming. If your house already has a pool, fine. If not, prepare for an investment of something like the equivalent of a first-class trip around the world or the purchase of a new Cadillac. A new swimming pool exercise we've just heard about is "water walking"—walking in the pool. The resistance of the water multiplies the effectiveness of your exercise.

In your neighborhood

Neighborhood exercise choices including walking, jogging, biking, and, for those who live in snowy country, cross-country skiing in winter. You can also look for a public swimming pool in your neighborhood. Some condo complexes allow nonresidents to use their pools for a membership fee.

In a fitness center or gym

Almost all modern fitness centers have aerobic exercise available as well as weights and Nautilus-style machines for muscle-strengthening exercises. At the L.A. Fitness gym where we go, the trainers want you to warm up for at least twenty minutes on the aerobic equipment before you begin your strength training workout. Not a bad idea, because a little of each is always better than a lot of either.

The advantage of the gym is that you can go in any weather and do a variety of exercises; the disadvantage is that at certain hours, especially early mornings and evenings, they are overcrowded and you have to waste time waiting to use the equipment. Ask the attendants which hours are the least popular and see if you can work your schedule around those times.

The other leading disadvantage is the cost. The initial fee can be as low as free if the company is running an advertised special or it could be up to $150. There is a monthly charge of maybe $25 to $50, depending on your neighborhood (high-rent areas charge the most); often family members can sign on together for lower rates. Be sure to investigate the company, as lots of scammy stuff goes on with some of these chains. The gym may go out of business after you've paid a big up-front fee, or it may sell out to another organization that won't honor your initial contract.

Now comes the big decision. You've picked your main workout location, so which particular sports are you going to go for? Here are some guidelines:

- Choose the exercises that most appeal to you.
- Choose the exercises you can do most often.
- Choose more than one exercise, especially if you're older, so that you can alternate them and give different muscles time to recoup between sessions.
- Choose aerobic exercise, but add some form of muscle-strengthening exercise. Sixty-five percent of the body's muscles are above the hips and most aerobic exercises do little to strengthen them.

- Choose some load-bearing exercise. For example, if swimming is your main thing, also do some activity in which you're on your feet. This is especially important for women because it helps avoid osteoporosis.

WALKING: SHOES AND SOCKS

VIRGINIA: That sounds like an ideal plan, but you know many of us will be lucky to get into *one* form of exercise. And some of us Type 2s need a little extra nudge to put us on the right track. Couldn't you give us at least a hint about which exercise would be the easiest and least likely to defeat us in the beginning?

JUNE AND BARBARA: That's exactly what we were hoping you would ask. The answer is clear and unequivocal: walking. To quote the albeit somewhat prejudiced author of a book on walking, Casey Meyers, "Walking is the most injury-free, sustainable, effective, complete exercise" there is. He also claims it uses more energy and burns more calories than running. Furthermore, Meyers proves via research that humans are biomechanically engineered to be walkers, not runners. As he puts it, "If God had meant humans to run, He would have given us the locomotion system of a horse."

Walking's our all-time favorite. Though we do other sports off and on, it's the activity we've most successfully woven into the fabric of our lives. It's a low-impact, lifetime exercise. You can do it fast (4 miles an hour) or slow (2 miles an hour). It's quick, convenient, and inexpensive. You can do it alone, with one other person, or in a group. Group and individual mallwalking programs are now available for people of all ages in some shopping centers. In our neighborhood, there are two walking tracks in two parks and we see people out doing their fitness walks at all hours of the day (except when it's 100 degrees outside).

Walking is also a perfect vacation sight-seeing activity. This year we spent ten days walking all over Florence and two weeks walking streets and roads and trails in the area around Montreux, Switzerland.

Walking is the least expensive exercise, especially compared to such equipment-intensive sports such as golfing, aerobics classes, tennis, and skiing. But there are a couple of things you do have to invest a bit of money in: shoes and socks. For a person with diabetes, choosing these isn't exactly a simple matter. We say this because of the amount of attention that must be paid to the legendary "diabetic foot." You find long lists of do's and don'ts about foot care in all diabetes manuals. We were surprised when one of our own books was indexed with a heading "diabetic foot," because no other part of the diabetic body was so listed. There was no entry for the diabetic thumb or ear. It's as if when you have diabetes, your Achilles heel is a whole Achilles foot. Virginia, here is where you come in. Can you explain why diabetic feet are different from ordinary feet?

VIRGINIA: Actually, diabetic feet start out like normal feet but suffer the effects of the disease as time goes by. When glucose levels stay above normal—over 180–200—year after year, two different problems add up to serious changes in the feet.

The first problem is the decrease in circulation that can occur because of diabetes. Excess glucose works to plug up your blood vessels. Poor circulation in your feet and legs means that they can't respond to the stress of a little sore by combating germs and infections. Your feet cannot heal the way normal feet do.

The second problem is the damage to nerves that high blood sugar can cause. When the nerves serving your feet and legs are damaged, they act like a faulty electrical circuit. First, you get static—tingling, strange shooting pains—and eventually numbness. This may seem like a relief after the tingling and pain, but it's very dangerous, because you don't know when you're getting the kind of excessive pressure that causes blisters, or you may be unaware that you've stepped on a tack. Eventually you could end up with structural deformities of the foot, because it is the nerves that keep the muscles stimulated to hold your feet in shape.

This is why diabetic feet need special tender loving care.

JUNE AND BARBARA: And that's the reason we're going to go into detail about purchasing shoes and socks. Not that everyone—with diabetes or not—who is an avid walker or jogger shouldn't be concerned about choosing the right foot attire. You can't enjoy walking unless your feet feel good both during and after. And it's not easy to make your selection these days since there is a proliferation of walking and running shoes and all the major brands have some new technology to hype. Something new comes along every day, and the buyer has to be wary.

Not only is there controversy about all this fancy technology, but there is little agreement about whether you should buy shoes designed specifically for walking or shoes specifically designed for running. We personally go for running shoes since the tread is usually more pronounced and therefore cushions and grips better. Robert Sweetgall says you should make sure that the shoes do not have flat bottoms. They should have a rocker profile; you ought to be able to see daylight under the toes and heels.

VIRGINIA: I have traded my Asics Gels for a pair of Rykas. My business partner (and exercise fanatic), Cathy, says they are designed especially for the female foot. I don't know about that, but they feel great and don't slip on my heels.

JUNE AND BARBARA: Then you agree with the experts who say that comfort is all. We advise people to go to a sports shoe shop, where the salespeople are often fanatical walkers or runners themselves and may know more and care more than the department store shoe salesperson. You should insist on a choice of several different brands and you should try each on and walk around a bit—even go outdoors and try them on the sidewalk—until you can decide on the most comfortable. Above all, do not settle for anything but your own size (some salespeople will try to peddle what they have in stock, even if it's a half-size too short or long or narrower or wider than you require). You should have a thumb width between the end of your toe and the end of the shoe.

And a word to women: Don't worry about looks. These are not things of beauty, but sports shoes are in style now all over America, so just change your thinking about what is attractive on your feet.

What are these ideally comfortable and well-fitting walking or running shoes going to cost? More than you'll want to pay for a pair for yourself (especially if you're a woman), but about what you would be willing to pay for a pair for your kid. Sixty to ninety dollars is not outrageous. The bad news is that when you get into walking 20 or so miles a week, you'll need to toss out the old and bring in the new every six months. As one sports shoe expert told us, you wouldn't want to drive around on worn-out tires with no tread. It's just as bad to walk around on worn-out shoes with no tread. One little money-saving tip is that sometimes you can pick up the previous model of a newly redesigned shoe at a lesser cost than the latest version. New models come on the market so frequently that the previous one is usually just as good structurally as the latest edition.

In addition to sport shoes, most comfortable brands of casual shoes, such as those made by Rockport and Ecco, can be used for walking, and they're particularly appropriate for city walking. In New York, the women have worked out a good compromise. They wear sport shoes—usually militantly and grubbily white ones to walk to work. Once they reach the office, they change into their corporate, go-to-meeting types.

Now for the socks. Seven or eight dollars a pair will buy you socks that will help prevent blisters and/or give you extra padding on the ball of the foot where you might have pain if your fat pad has grown thin over the years or if you tend to build up calluses. As verified by a study in *Diabetes Medicine*, this extra padding may also prevent diabetic foot problems by reducing the pressure on the vulnerable parts of the foot.

Some of our favorite brands include Double Lay'R Socks (for blister prevention; very soft); Seamfree Socks (no seams to rub and create blisters); TheraSock, another double sock system that reduces friction; and Thor-Lo athletic socks, which have extra knitting at the heel and ball areas. Thor-Lo makes many kinds of athletic socks (tennis, golf, aerobics) so make sure you get the walking socks. These brands are usually available in sports shoe shops and by mail order (Double Lay'R and Seamfree: 1-800-973-9939; TheraSock: 1-800-433-2489; Thor-Lo: 1-800-457-2256).

VIRGINIA: I'd like to add that when buying your shoes you should wear your padded socks. And I like stores whose salespeople know how to fit you the old-fashioned way. Remember when you were a kid, the salesperson would feel the shoe and tell you whether or not it fit? If you have "at risk" feet, you have diminished sensation and you can't trust your feet to tell you how well the shoe fits. It's not worth saving a few dollars at a discount self-serve shoe store and losing a foot!

Now how about telling us how walking becomes an aerobic exercise in the sense that it strengthens the heart and helps control blood pressure?

JUNE AND BARBARA: You have to walk fast enough to increase your heart rate (number of beats per minute) to at least 65 percent of its maximum rate. That means you have to walk a mile in about seventeen minutes. The standard way of figuring your maximum heart rate is easy: Subtract your age from the number 220. For instance, if you're fifty-five, the formula is 220 – 55 = 165 beats per minute. (You definitely don't want to reach that rate during exercise.) Then take 65 percent of 165 and you get 107 beats per minute. That's your "target rate," but most of you will have to consider your age and physical condition and approach that target slowly. Also, remember Covert Bailey's caution that this formula may not apply to you individually, so you might want to check with your doctor.

To monitor your pulse, check it before, during, and after exercise. Using your fingertips, find your pulse at your wrist (inside) or at the carotid artery underneath your jawbone at the left side of your neck. Count for 10 seconds and multiply by 6 to get your heartbeats per minute. (Our guru Covert Bailey prefers that you count for 6 seconds and multiply by 10; this does make multiplying easier, but it's harder to count for exactly 6 seconds because it's such a short time.)

The goal is to keep your heart rate at its target of 60 percent for about twenty to thirty minutes at a time. Only a sustained, uninterrupted effort for this amount of time can condition your heart. This kind of continuous, rhythmical exercise that uses the muscles of the lower body is what's called aerobic exercise. Walking, of course, is only one of many such exercises. You can choose from bicycling, swimming, jogging, aerobic dancing, roller skating, jumping rope, and others.

VIRGINIA: I get the picture, and I know you start out slowly, with your doctor's approval, if you haven't been doing much of anything in the exercise line. As far as diabetes is concerned, I have to recommend also that you not only monitor your heart rate, but you also monitor your blood sugar if you take pills or insulin, especially insulin. Your blood sugar should be at least 150 before you start your exercise session. If it's less, eat a snack before starting. If it's over 250, there's another factor to consider. There may not be adequate insulin on board to handle the increased demand for fuel that will occur with exercise, and your blood sugar will go up even higher.

In helping patients set up an exercise program, I always explain that they should do their exercise for at least twenty to thirty minutes at a time at least three or four times a week. It should be done at a level that feels somewhat difficult, but not so strenuously that you feel out of breath. And above all, don't exceed your target heart range.

STRENGTH TRAINING

JUNE AND BARBARA: We hate to remind you that aerobic activity is not the end of the exercise program anymore. All the experts claim now, and we certainly go along with them, that aerobics alone are not enough. You must also do some strength training.

VIRGINIA: You mean pumping iron? Who wants big biceps and show-off muscles? I certainly don't want to look like Popeye and not many of my patients do either.

JUNE AND BARBARA: Don't get us wrong. We don't either. What is being advocated for health benefits has nothing to do with professional body building. Strength training is done by lifting hand-held weights or using weight machines like Nautilus. It's been shown that this kind of training retards the aging process—and you can't knock that. It can make a ninety-year-old as strong as a fifty-year-old. But the biggest news is that besides reducing the risk of getting diabetes, it improves insulin sensitivity, and that should make it especially popular with all Type 2s.

VIRGINIA: Come to think of it, it has another great advantage: It improves the body's proportion of muscle to fat, and this really counts from a health standpoint. If your body has a high percentage of fat, it does not require as many calories to preserve that fat. The result is that when you eat extra calories, the body stores them with all that other fat. This is not good news unless you're preparing for a famine. So by converting fat to muscle you can change your metabolism so that you burn more calories. This, of course, helps solve weight problems.

JUNE AND BARBARA: That's why some health professionals think recommended weight should be determined by measuring the proportion of fat and lean tissue. They don't consider the old height-weight tables good guides. We admit that if we followed what's considered normal weight on those tables, we'd be total tubs. But many people feel the federal governments's new standard for healthy weight (established in 1998 by the National Institutes of Health) has gone too far the other way. This defines anyone with a BMI—body-mass index (a formula used to estimate body fat)— of more than 25 as overweight. The definition of "obese" is a BMI greater than 30.

According to these definitions, 55 percent of adult Americans would be considered overweight.

Dr. Xavier Pi-Sunyer, who heads the NIH task force, was quoted in the *Wall Street Journal* as conceding that "the scientific literature doesn't prove conclusively that people with BMIs over 25 will have a shorter life span—*unless they have another condition such as diabetes.*" (Italics are ours!) He also said that the literature doesn't show that people who are overweight according to the new standards are at increased risk of developing health problems, such as *diabetes* and high blood pressure. (Again the italics are ours.)

This is likely to turn into one of those extended health wrangles until a new controversy comes along to take its place. In the meantime, if you want to check yourself out against this new standard, here's how you do it. (This will make a great parlor game at your next social gathering.) You divide your body weight in kilograms by your height in meters squared. Since this is tough for Americans, since we don't know our dimensions in the metric system, you can also just multiply your weight in pounds by 703, and then divide the result by your height in inches. Then divide that result by your height a second time.

$$\text{BMI} = \frac{\text{weight in kilograms (total pounds} \div 2.2)}{\text{height in meters}^2 \ (\sqrt{\text{total inches}} \times 2.5 \div 100)}$$

If you don't like how this turns out, you can spend some more time and some money by getting yourself weighed underwater using a hydrosensitomer. Since fat floats and muscle sinks, the heavier you are underwater, the better. (It's the opposite of the situation on land.) But in your heart of hearts, you probably already know if you're overweight or obese and should do something about it. Women, however, have a tendency to think to think of themselves as overweight ("I've just got to lose 10 pounds!") when they're not, and men have a tendency to think they're not overweight ("I'm just husky.") when they are. This test, which is the most accurate, could help people toward a more realistic assessment than working from a chart.

VIRGINIA: Okay, let's get back to muscle building. You've made your point. How do you get going on it and how do you learn how to do it?

JUNE AND BARBARA: It's not as hard as you may think. You don't even have to grunt. In fact, you shouldn't exert yourself that much. And you only have to do it about twice a week. We usually alternate it with our walking exercise, as you don't want to do strength training two days in a row. Your muscles like to rest.

VIRGINIA: Well, I don't have a gym near where I live. Does that mean I can't do muscle strengthening?

JUNE AND BARBARA: No, it just means you do it at home using free weights. The main problem with that is, unless your diabetes center has an exercise therapist on staff, you'll have to find one to visit or you'll have to buy one of the better books on weight lifting. Two of these are *Designing Resistance Training Programs* by S. J. Fleck and W. J. Kraemer (Champaign, Ill.: Human Kinetics Books, 1987); and *Lift Your Way to Youthful Fitness* by Jerry Todd and Jan Todd (Boston: Little, Brown, 1985).

We're lucky because there are plenty of gyms in Southern California and when we're free to go at uncrowded hours we can get an excellent workout in a short time. There's something motivating about a gym. A "Personal Health" column in the *Los Angeles Times* about sticking with exercise revealed that women need social support to adopt and maintain an exercise program, while men are motivated by a favorable environment. In a gym you do fraternize with the other exercisers and the environment is more than favorable, because you can't do anything but exercise while you're there. And we find it fun to learn to use the fancy new fitness machines. Our gym has Nautilus and Cybex equipment. The latter are easy to set, smooth to use, and make you feel like a real pro.

When you join a gym you usually get at least one complimentary lesson with a trainer who designs a program just for you. But you have to watch out when signing on, as gyms are now a big business and a very competitive one, and some firms have indulged in fraudulent activities, like signing up hundreds of people and then going out of business or charging excessive start-up fees with the hope that you'll sign on and then drop out within a few months. All have aggressive sales staffs to push you into signing a contract. So beware; you've been warned.

VIRGINIA: Can you give us a brief glimpse of what you actually do during a workout? Some people have never been inside a gym. And are there any cautions for persons with diabetes?

JUNE AND BARBARA: You're supposed to work at least eight or ten different muscle groups and do one set of each exercise. A set is ten to twelve repetitions. For instance, we do abdominal, back extension, arm curl, rowing, chest press, lateral pulldown, lateral rise, leg extension, leg curl, and hip adduction. (Those terms are probably mysterious to you, because you have to see the machines to know what they mean.) The load you set the machine for (in 5- or 10-pound increments) has to be light enough so that you can lift it at least eight times before your muscles fatigue. If you can lift it more than fifteen times, it's too light. You work up to about thirty repetitions and then you go on to the next heavier weight.

VIRGINIA: How do you keep from injuring yourself? I've known people who strained muscles in gyms.

JUNE AND BARBARA: Experts William Evans, chief of the Human Physiology Laboratory at the Human Nutrition Research Center on Aging at Tufts University, and Michael Preuss, fitness director at Cooper Aerobics Center in Dallas, give these cautions:

- Lift slowly, avoiding jerky or "explosive" movements. Lifting a weight should take two or three seconds; lowering it should take about the same amount of time.

- Ask a trainer in the health club to demonstrate proper breathing technique.
- Ask your doctor's advice or get an examination before beginning, especially if you're older or have diabetes or high blood pressure.
- Don't go overboard. An every-other-day program works best.

We would alter that last caution to once or twice a week. And if you have proliferative diabetic retinopathy (a disease of the retina), weight training is a great risk. In fact, get permission from your ophthalmologist if you have even moderate retinopathy. Also talk to your doctor if you have chronic hypertension.

VIRGINIA: I think I need to go rest now. Do you have any final words about exercise?

JUNE AND BARBARA: We have a final story about weight lifting that we know you'd like to hear.

We read an article in the May 1992 *Diabetes Forecast* that profiled Ron Gillembardo of Las Vegas. Ron was diagnosed with Type 2 diabetes in 1982 when he was thirty-eight years old. His blood sugar was 500 and he tipped the scales at 360 pounds. He started working out with weights and he just happened to excel at it. In less than two years, he lost nearly 100 pounds and he got off insulin and onto pills. He kept working out with weights two hours a day, five days a week.

In 1989 Ron began power lifting in competitions. He won almost every competition he entered and became the world record holder in the 710-pound lift. At the age of forty-three he qualified for the 1992 Olympic Games in Barcelona. He is the oldest weight lifter ever to compete in the Olympics.

Now doesn't that make you want to get out there and see what kind of prizes you can win with exercise? The best prize, of course, will be your wonderful diabetes control and your new self-esteem.

CHAPTER 4

FOOD, DIET, NUTRITION:

The "Only More So" Disease

People with diabetes are not that different from the rest of the population. When you come right down to it, for optimum health, a person with Type 2 diabetes needs to do what anyone else should do—only more so. Everybody needs to be on an exercise program; so does the person with diabetes—only more so. All inhabitants of the modern world need to learn how to handle personal and work and societal stresses; so does the person with diabetes—only more so.

Never does the "only more so factor" apply more strongly than in the area of diet. Everyone needs to follow a healthy diet, but diabetic people need to follow a diet that is even more healthy than the average person's. But, the big question these days is: What is a healthy diet? Reports issued by the U.S. Surgeon General, National Institutes of Health, American Heart Association, American Dietetic Association, American Medical Association, as well as battalions of medical and dietary experts (and self-proclaimed experts) all tell us the right diet to follow. But they point in so many different—

and constantly changing—directions that we often don't know which way to go. Our newsletter, *The Diabetic Reader*, includes a regular column called "The Fickle Finger of Food Facts." In each issue we report the new pronouncements that negate the previous ones: Coffee, which was a bad thing one year, is declared harmless the next; we were told to cut back drastically on salt for a period, and then suddenly we were warned that many people weren't getting enough salt, causing them to have a sodium deficiency; at the urging of Linus Pauling and others we loaded up on vitamin C for cold prevention and antioxidant benefits, then came an assertion that vitamin C has pro-oxidant as well as antioxidant effects, and therefore could cause genetic damage if taken in large doses. Everybody is totally confused—and people with diabetes are even more so.

We're going to do our best to alleviate some of diabetes dietary confusion, but it won't be easy. Just as in Supreme Court decisions, we have a majority opinion and a minority opinion. The conservative majority says that the best diet for Type 2s is high in complex carbohydrates and fiber and low in fat. The so-called radical minority believes that a low-carbohydrate diet with more protein, and therefore fat, is the answer. Between the three of us we'll try—just like attorneys—to defend both positions and explain some of the secondary—but still important—dietary considerations along the way. When you discover the diet or, more likely, dietary variations that work best for you, you'll find that before long you'll look and feel as healthy, vital, and vibrant as your nondiabetic contemporaries.

—*June and Barbara*

SWIMMING IN THE CONSERVATIVE MAINSTREAM: THE LOW-FAT, HIGH-CARBOHYDRATE, HIGH-FIBER DIET

JUNE AND BARBARA: When people are diagnosed with Type 2 diabetes, they're usually told that with a little bit of luck they can probably control their blood sugar level simply by changing their diet and adding regular exercise. This is a comforting thought, compared with taking blood-sugar-lowering pills or injections of insulin, but is it true?

VIRGINIA: Yes, Type 2 diabetes can be managed with diet and weight loss in many cases. Statistics tell us that among people with Type 2 diabetes, 40 percent control their diabetes with pills, and about 35 percent with insulin. This means that less than 25 percent are controlling blood sugar with diet and exercise alone—usually a code for "doing nothing" because too often the person with Type 2 has not been referred to a nutritionist or an exercise program. Does this mean that two-thirds of all Type 2s are bad people who don't follow a proper diet? No, these statistics probably reflect the evolution of the disease.

Initially, the disease is manifested primarily in insulin resistance and is amenable to treatment with diet and exercise. As the insulin deficiency becomes more severe, the need for oral agents and insulin increases. Eventually, when the insulin deficiency and excessive liver glucose production outstrip the pills' ability to control blood sugars, insulin becomes essential.

When I was at the Presbyterian Diabetes Center, we suggested what we call the Fast Fast to help many people get their blood sugars into control quickly, or to get off medications if they're already using them.

The Fast Fast is not really a fast. It's a fast from carbohydrates only. (All foods are composed of various combinations of carbohydrate, protein, and fat; carbohydrates are sugars and starches and they usually account for about 50 percent of what we eat.) On the Fast Fast you can eat as much salad with low-fat dressing as you want. You eat at least one small meat serving a day, baked, broiled, or boiled, and all the sugar-free gelatin you can stand, any color. You can also have all the sugar-free sodas, coffee, and tea you want, but on top of that you should be sure to drink at least eight large glasses of water a day.

THE "FAST FAST"

JUNE AND BARBARA: How do most people feel while on the Fast Fast?

VIRGINIA: They usually don't feel bad at all. What happens is that they get a headache the first day and then they're not even hungry after that.

We always have people on the Fast Fast test their blood sugar at least twice a day, because blood sugars can drop precipitously. People on insulin or pills will need a health professional to coach them so they know how to decrease their medication in anticipation of the lowering blood sugars. Otherwise they might get too low and run out and attack a donut shop or something. To get off the pills or insulin and achieve the goal glucose level takes three to five days. Then you start adding carbohydrates . . . slowly. First add low-carbohydrate green vegetables such as green beans, broccoli, spinach, and the like. Even though they're green, peas are almost pure starch, so don't add them yet. Avocados are high in fat, so don't add them. Next try adding toast for breakfast, then maybe a potato at dinner. In other words, gradually add one carbohydrate at a time to see the effect on your blood sugar.

Let me tell you about Mary Jane, a nurse who works nights and has had Type 2 diabetes for eight or ten years. She was one of the students in a nursing course I was teaching for the University of Phoenix in Albuquerque. She introduced herself, rather proudly, as a "noncompliant" diabetic. (At the time, she was unaware of what I did for a living.) She was a typical picture of a person with diabetes who had been blamed for her disease for so long that she pinned the "noncompliant" label on herself before anyone else had a chance to. She was 75 pounds overweight, taking large amounts of insulin, but still her blood glucose levels usually ran from 200 to 400. She felt bad all the time and she felt helpless to stop her cycle of overeating and poor control. Worst of all, she believed her problems were all her own fault.

After we had known each other for a few weeks, Mary Jane

came up to me after class and described how she would wake up with low blood sugar every afternoon and eat the house down for the rest of the evening. Then she'd go to work at 10:30 P.M. and feel awful. (Her insulin regimen was the same as if she had been on a day schedule.) I asked her to let me know when she was ready to get off insulin and I would help her.

She waited a few weeks before she brought up the subject. I told her how to do the Fast Fast, lowering her insulin as her blood glucose levels came down. (Since she was a nurse, she could be trusted to handle this on her own.) She called me on the weekend to complain that she felt awful. She wasn't used to having blood glucose levels in the normal range; of course, she felt entirely different from when she was 200 to 300 all the time. But even though she felt bad, boy, was she excited and happy because *she was off insulin!*

She had an appointment with her doctor for that next week. I told her to ask him for a prescription for an oral hypoglycemic agent so that if her blood glucose levels started going up a little as she gradually added back carbohydrate food, she would have a safety net. We also spent a great deal of time talking about how to eat light, low-fat meals and about starting to exercise.

Her doctor was shocked that she was off insulin and that her fasting blood glucose was down to 185. (She would get lower than that throughout the day, but that pesky liver would pop it up during the night, and that's why she needed the pills.) The doctor suggested she go back on insulin, and Mary Jane rightly replied, "Remember what my blood glucose level was when I was on insulin?" On top of that, she was now 12 pounds lighter. By taking Diabeta pills (she calls them Diabetter) and getting back on carbohydrates, she is keeping her blood glucose levels between 100 and 200 and has lost a total of 35 pounds. She's exercising at least three hours a week and is feeling better than she has in years.

JUNE AND BARBARA: The Fast Fast sounds like a miracle cure, but Mary Jane had had diabetes for eight or ten years. Does the Fast Fast work equally well for newly diagnosed diabetics?

VIRGINIA: Yes, I have another success story for you that proves it. I met Nick in the hospital. His doctor had hospitalized him as a newly diagnosed diabetic, although most endocrinologists, instead of putting patients in the hospital, let us at the Presbyterian Diabetes Center do their initial training and glucose control as outpatients. Nick, a good-looking though chubby Hispanic guy about thrity-five years old, is a computer operator who leads a pretty sedentary life. He had gone to the doctor with symptoms of excess urination, excess thirst, and generally feeling awful. He suspected diabetes, because most of the people in his family over the age of sixty had the disease. He had not lost large amounts of weight during this period of illness. In fact, he was about 50 pounds overweight.

The doctor had him on 70/30 insulin (NPH and Regular pre-mixed in a vial) and wanted him to get a blood glucose testing meter. I was to teach him how to use the meter. His blood sugars were still moderately high, in the 200s. I told him that it would be useful for him to be on insulin, because otherwise his health insurance would not pay for a meter. But I promised him that we could get him off insulin pronto, whenever he was ready. He looked at me as if I were crazy. I think the doctor must have told him I *was* crazy, because we didn't see him again at the Center for a few months.

He finally decided to come to our eight-week course. He was still on insulin, but his dose was lower. He had lost about 10 pounds, because his wife was following the diet guidelines given to them in the hospital. When he showed up in class, he asked me about getting off insulin. I said, "Sure, Nick, whenever you're ready." I knew it wouldn't be difficult, because he was on so little insulin—about 16 units in the morning and 10 units at night. For a guy weighing over 200 pounds, if he really needed insulin, it would have taken a lot more than that. Besides, when you're young and brand-new to diabetes, the Fast Fast works especially well.

He started on the Fast and in a few days was normoglycemic (another word for euglycemic) and off insulin.

JUNE AND BARBARA: We're happy to hear you talk about people getting off insulin. There's a terrible rumor going around that once you start taking insulin you have to take it forever. One Type 2 woman, who had always been controlled with diet and exercise, wrote and told us of a terrifying experience for her. She had been hospitalized for surgery and the stress caused her blood sugars to go up. When her doctors told her they were going to give her some insulin to bring it down, she fainted dead away. That was because she thought she was going to be on insulin for the rest of her life. After her recovery, her blood sugar went back down and she could again control her diabetes without insulin. "But," she complained, "why did I have to go through that when it wasn't necessary? Why didn't someone explain to me that this was just a temporary thing?" Why indeed? Let's hear it for letting the patient know what's going on! But how about Nick? Is he still off insulin?

VIRGINIA: Yes, he's continued to keep his blood glucose in control with diet and exercise. He has a nice blood glucose meter to keep track of it, thanks to his health insurance. If Nick can keep losing weight, he'll probably be able to control his diabetes for many years with diet and exercise. This is not to say that the disease was solely caused by his diet, his obesity, or his sedentary lifestyle. Those factors were certainly not in his favor, but we know lots of guys just like Nick—overweight, sedentary lifestyle—who don't have diabetes. Remember, Type 2 diabetes is a genetic disease, not a character flaw!

LOW-FAT LIFESTYLE

JUNE AND BARBARA: Many people newly diagnosed with diabetes are sent by their doctors to a dietitian. In our opinion, this is definitely the way to go. People think the dietitian will tell them to get off sugar forever, but instead the talk is mostly about fat. We also noticed that at the Diabetes Network you have a teaching manual that recommends the "low-fat lifestyle." Why is fat such a big deal for Type 2 diabetics?

VIRGINIA: You're right in noticing that fat is a big deal. In fact, it may be the biggest deal for the Type 2s, whose bodies actually have a preference for fat as a fuel source. Nondiabetics normally use glucose as their fuel of preference. The glucose is shuttled into the muscle cells via the cells' receptors thanks to insulin "opening the door." Glucose is used strictly as fuel; fat goes into storage.

Now let's say you're a Type 2 and your muscle cell receptors don't work so well. They can't make use of the insulin to get the glucose into the cell. One thing Mother Nature did for us as a safety valve was to give us the ability to use fatty acids as well as glucose for fuel. So when they can't get to the glucose, your muscles can use fatty acids as their fuel to keep going.

When you eat a meal with 50 percent of the calories from fat, here come the two fuels, fat and glucose, floating down the bloodstream to meet your muscles. The muscles would actually prefer the glucose, but what will they do if they can't get the glucose in? They grab the fat and use it as their fuel and leave the glucose floating around. That's why you end up with high blood sugar after a high-fat meal.

This is not the way it works in people who don't have diabetes. In a normal person, fat goes straight into storage and doesn't raise the blood sugar. Fat is not sugar. It doesn't even convert to blood sugar except under extreme circumstances.

But the Type 2 diabetic has high blood sugar because his or her body used the fat for fuel instead of the glucose; the insulin level is high as well because the pancreas is making more insulin to deal with the high blood sugar. Now the insulin is going to store the glucose as fat. So into storage it goes, and the Type 2 gains more weight.

A recent article in the *Obesity Journal* (I was asked to be the centerfold but I declined) looked at a large number of people with and without diabetes and measured their body fat levels and then tracked their eating habits over a long period of time. The researchers noted two things. One, thin people and fat people eat about the same amount of calories (this was already a well-known fact). Two, thin people eat less than 30 percent of their calories as fat, and fat people eat more than 30 percent of their calories as fat. This is the big difference.

So can we cut our fat consumption to 10, 20, or 25 percent of our calories and lose weight? The jury is not in on this yet, but it is certainly looking like the way to go for some people. For the person with diabetes, this is neither as easy nor as difficult as it sounds. If you cut the fat, you have to add carbohydrates in order to have enough calories. To prevent the high-carbohydrate diet from raising your blood glucose levels, you have to be careful to add lots of fiber, because fiber slows down the entry of glucose into the blood and also makes you more sensitive to your own insulin. If in combination with a low-fat and high-fiber diet you also get plenty of exercise, you'll not only lose weight, but you'll be the healthiest you could ever be! This is what we call the "low-fat lifestyle," and if it's beginning to sound familiar, it should. It is the recommendation for a healthy heart, cancer prevention, and good health in general.

We advise people not to think of this as a diet. People who go on diets go off diets. We ask our patients to go on a lifeplan. Eating less than 20 to 30 percent fat requires some fundamental changes, but if you give yourself plenty of the carbohydrates that you love, you'll feel great and not get into the "deprivation mode," a surefire way to blow your diet!

JUNE AND BARBARA: Many experts agree that fat, not carbohydrate, is the real enemy. Avoiding fat is the cornerstone of the successful Pritikin weight-loss (and health-gain!) diet and of the Martin Katahn T-Factor diet. It's also basic in Dr. James Anderson's high-carbohydrate, high-fiber, low-fat diet (HCF diet), which allows only 9 percent calories as fat but so improves insulin sensitivity in Type 2 diabetics that in one study the diet resulted in 52 percent of overweight Type 2s being taken off insulin completely.

Now tell us exactly how you follow a low-fat diet.

VIRGINIA: Get obsessed with fat! Look for it everywhere. Get a calorie and nutrient counter paperback at the bookstore and start looking at every label of every food product you consider buying. Any more than 5 grams of fat in a serving is probably too much. To find out how many grams of fat you can have, estimate your total daily calories—for example, 1,600. Now multiply by 20 percent to find out how many calories of fat you can have. This would be 320. Now divide those calories by 9 to determine the grams of fat you can have (each gram of fat has 9 calories). The answer is 36. (That's seven fat exchanges if you use the American Diabetes Association's exchange lists). Thirty-six grams of fat are plenty to keep you dietarily happy.

Look at breakfast, for example. Skim milk has no fat. (I use 1/2 percent milk to avoid the transparent look of skim, but that's only 1 gram of fat per cup, whereas low-fat milk contains 5 grams a cup.) Cheerios (and many other cereals, hot or cold) are fat free. A banana is fat free. Hey, this is really easy . . . no problem.

Now how about lunch? You were going to eat macaroni and cheese? Think again. A typical serving (about twice the recommended amount) has 35 grams of fat—your whole day's supply! You really have to watch cheeses. In fact, most cheese recipes—you know, a little leftover this and that and cover it with about a cup of grated cheddar and voilà, a masterpiece—are high in fat. All those years we watched the Kraft show on Sunday nights and believed that cheese was a health food—and now you find out it was all a lie! We should have known that anyone who would put a glop of mayonnaise on Jell-O would lie about cheese, too!

So what are some good choices for lunch? Try a baked potato topped with low-fat cottage cheese and chives. Tastes better than sour cream. How about pasta with a tomato and mushroom sauce with no meat? You should keep the pasta down to 1 cup. If that still leaves you feeling hungry, add a salad with fat-free dressing and a vegetable, such as zucchini or green beans. If you want meat, make it skinless chicken, fish, or a very small serving of lean red meat. You'll have to be very careful about eating meat. In many cases, half the calories in a meat serving come from fat. Put another way, the quarter-pound hamburger patty (3 ounces cooked) has 10 to 15 grams of fat—and that's without cheese or mayonnaise.

Dinner? Well, you must be getting the idea by now. Just get out that fat gram counter and you'll be safe.

JUNE AND BARBARA: It's really important to have a fat gram counter and understand clearly where fat lurks in food. A lot of people just don't get it. During the 1992 Republican convention, we heard a radio interview from a Houston barbecue place that was a favorite of then-President Bush since back when he was in the oil business in that city. Bush had stopped by to eat while he was in town for the convention. The interviewer asked the owner of the place what Bush had selected for his meal. She said that he had barbecued beef, barbecued ribs, and hot links with cole slaw. She said that normally he would have had baked beans instead of the cole slaw, but he had told her he was on a low-fat diet. Wowee! The only thing that might possibly have been low fat in that place were the baked beans—assuming they weren't loaded with bacon or ham.

To keep you from inadvertently living off the fat of the land, we'd like to suggest a few fat gram counters so you can run right out and buy one while you're fired up on the idea. There's a huge choice, but we'll only list the ones you're most likely to find in your local bookstore.

> *The Corinne T. Netzer Fat Gram Counter* (Dell, $4.50)
>
> *Fat & Fiber in Your Food* by Art Ulene, M.D. (Avery Publishing Group, $5.95)
>
> *The Fat Counter* by Annette Natow and Jo-Ann Heslin (Pocket Books, $5.99)
>
> *The T-Factor Fat Gram Counter* by Jamie Pope-Cordle and Martin Katahn (Norton, $2.50)
>
> *The Vest Pocket Fat Counter* by Susan Podell (Doubleday, $2.99)

(Note: If you have trouble finding these, write to us at 5623 Matilija Ave., Van Nuys, CA 91401 and request a *Diabetic Reader,* where you'll find reviews, excerpts, and ordering information for important books on diabetes.)

When you come right down to it, just how easy—or hard—is it for most people to follow such a low-fat diet?

VIRGINIA: Take it from one who's doing it: It's not easy to get out there and live in the real world on a really low-fat diet. Temptation is ubiquitous. The first rule of thumb is: If it's fried, forget it! Cheese is a real no-no. This is the most painful part for me. I love cheese! At home I use the fat-free or low-fat cheese slices (Kraft Free, Lite Line, and Alpine Lace are good ones) although they're a little salty for my taste, because I also cut down on salt. There are a few dishes that you need a little bit of cheese for, and these nonfat or low-fat varieties do the trick. They even melt nicely.

Another thing I really miss is mayonnaise. There are some good low-fat mayonnaises such as Lite Hellmans, which has half the fat of regular mayo, but even so it has 5 grams of fat per serving. Kraft makes a fat-free mayo, but as far as taste goes—yuck! I have discovered that I can buy some extremely low-fat dressings. I've found one with parmesan and garlic (boy, is that good!) and I use that mixed with tuna to make a tuna sandwich. On turkey or chicken sandwiches I use mustard, which is totally fat free.

How are you going to eat a potato without any fat on it? Besides low-fat cottage cheese with chives or green onion, try salsa. It gives the potato a really nice flavor.

RESTAURANT DINING

JUNE AND BARBARA: It's one thing when you're at home and in total control of the situation, but how about when you eat out? Eating in a restaurant is the hardest part of any diet—especially a low-fat one. Maybe you could give us a few tips on how you handle that.

VIRGINIA: Well, living in New Mexico as I do, my favorite food when dining out is our wonderful New Mexican cuisine. A typical

New Mexican food is enchiladas. They dip a tortilla in oil, then in chile (a sauce of red chile, not like Texas chili), they put cheese in it and fold it over, then they pour green chile over it and add more cheese—plenty of cheese. They also serve a lot of refried beans. The classic way to make refried beans is to start with pinto beans and add a cup or two of lard or bacon drippings.

My favorite restaurant, however, prepares their beans with no fat. They're nothing but cooked pinto beans mashed up. They taste just as good as the refried ones with all the fat—maybe even better since you feel so virtuous when you eat them. Of course, I don't order the enchiladas. I order off the à la carte menu and pick fat-free dishes. For instance, they have an excellent dish called Potatoes Garcia. It's just sliced potatoes cooked down until they're real soft, with cilantro and a touch of green chile added. Boy, are they good! No fat and wonderful flavor. I get a big tortilla and eat the beans and potatoes mixed up with a little green chile. Green chile sauce has little or no fat. You can be selective like this in any restaurant. When you order fish, ask them to grill or broil it and leave off the fat. Leave off the sauce, too. Most restaurants are happy to do that for you.

When I go into a restaurant and order a meal that includes a piece of meat that is much larger than I need, I know I'll eat it all if it's on my plate, so I ask my husband to split the entree with me. We each order our own potato and salad. That way I'll be quite satisfied with a serving of 2 or 3 ounces of meat.

JUNE AND BARBARA: We handle that too-large protein serving in a different way. We each order a full portion but take half of it home in a doggie bag. It's not too hard to resist the temptation to eat all of it if you know the leftovers will save you the trouble of shopping for and fixing a protein course at home the next night.

You can ask for doggie bags even in the best restaurants. We have a friend who is very socially prominent and has gone to the fanciest of private finishing schools. She now works as a volunteer at UCLA giving conversation classes to newly arrived foreign students. They ask her questions about experiences they've had that were confusing or upsetting to them. One Korean girl told our friend she was out to dinner with her boyfriend and at the end of the meal the waiter asked her if she wanted a doggie bag. She said, "I was so frightened! I didn't know what to say or do." Our friend explained what a doggie bag is and assured the student that she should never hesitate to ask for one because everybody does it and it's a perfectly correct thing to do. If she says it's OK, it must be!

VIRGINIA: Another good tip is to ask for the doggie bag at the beginning of the meal. Put half of your meat portion in it, and then you won't be tempted to eat the whole portion on your plate. Most of us have found that we must play lots of little games with ourselves to make our diets work. One trick is to focus on what you *can* have. And what you can have makes a wonderful life. You can feel good and you can have health. Don't focus on what it is you can't have, because that's a racket that will get you into trouble.

JUNE AND BARBARA: Some people who are genuine fatophobes may want to know if it's OK to eliminate all fat in an individual meal.

VIRGINIA: It's very difficult to totally eliminate 100 percent of the fat, although it's not impossible. You'll find, though, that if you eat a fat-free meal it's also probably virtually a protein-free meal and that means you'll get a pretty steep glucose rise after the meal. As I suggested previously, if you're on insulin, you can learn to cover the carbohydrate with your insulin dose. For most people, the formula is 1 unit of Regular insulin (fast acting) or Humalog for each 10 grams of carbohydrate. You can do that and then do a one-hour after-meal blood sugar reading to determine your own formula for covering food with insulin. Another tip when you're going to eat a high-carb meal is to take the regular insulin at least forty-five minutes before the meal so that the insulin will peak with the food.

I would like to comment, though, that no one would want to entirely eliminate fat 100 percent of the time because there are some incredibly important vitamins that we get from fat. These are the so-called fat soluble vitamins A, D, E, and K. Vitamin E is very important for keeping our skin soft and wrinkle free (as if that were possible!). It's also important for healing and we wouldn't want to slow that down. If you eat a normal diet of a little bit of meat here and there, use some olive oil once in a while on a salad, and have some dairy products (skim milk is fortified with vitamin D), you'll be safe on these vitamins. Also, remember that not all fats are "bad" fats.

JUNE AND BARBARA: You mean there is such a thing as "good" fat?

VIRGINIA: Yes, the monounsaturated fats are good for us. These are fats from olive oil, canola oil, peanut oil, and avocados. They still have 9 calories per gram but contribute to a healthy heart.

BINGE EATING

JUNE AND BARBARA: Jane Brody, health columnist for *The New York Times*, recently wrote a column about a new category of eating disorder, distinct from anorexia or bulimia and far more common than either of these. It's called "binge eating disorder," and accounts for a large proportion of seriously overweight Americans who repeatedly try to lose weight but fail. You've probably met hundreds of diabetics who fit this description. If binge eating disorder is their problem, they indulge in frequent, uncontrolled, and often hours-long eating episodes during which they may devour more than 2,000 calories. Psychologist Richard R. Rubin calls these "search and consume missions." Unlike people with bulimia, they do not attempt to purge their bodies of the excess calories by inducing vomiting or taking laxatives. They simply gain weight.

According to Dr. Robert L. Spitzer, who proposed that this disorder be included in the official manual of psychiatric diagnoses so that insurance would reimburse for its treatment, binge eaters tend to be depressed, anxious, or suffering other psychological disturbances much more than other people with comparable weight problems. Here are the criteria to identify the condition:

- Recurrent episodes of bingeing and the sense that the eating is out of control.
- Episodes occur at least twice a week on average, for six months or longer.
- The behavior causes marked distress.
- Binges involve at least three of these actions: eating much more rapidly than usual; eating to uncomfortable fullness; eating large amounts of food even when not hungry; eating alone out of embarrassment; feelings of disgust or guilt.

Unfortunately, going on a diet does not solve this problem; in fact, drastic dieting may trigger bingeing behavior. Overeaters Anonymous is a good form of group therapy for bingers. In fact, Dr. Spitzer's study found that 71 percent of participants in Overeaters Anonymous met his diagnostic criteria for binge eating disorder.

From your experience with seriously overweight diabetics, would you say that many of them have this psychological problem? If so, will treating it put them on the road to weight loss?

VIRGINIA: I'm sure that Dr. Spitzer is onto something here. I frequently encounter patients who use the very words, "My eating is out of control." There is one more stimulus that he hasn't noted that I feel may be very significant for a Type 2. As you proceed down the merry path of Type 2 diabetes—highly insulin resistant, making excessive amounts of insulin to control your blood glucose, but even so, only partially controlling it—your blood glucose goes up incrementally. In other words, you can sort of control your blood glucose, but if it goes up due to a dietary indiscretion—such as if you "accidentally" ate a chocolate bunny for Easter—your body cannot bring it back down and you will stay at the higher level. This is the phenomenon we've called glucose toxicity. It is a condition where your insulin works better at normal range glucoses. It also takes a lot more insulin to conquer a high blood glucose than to maintain a normal range.

JUNE AND BARBARA: June can certainly verify this. If her blood sugar is in the low 200s, it takes a supplement of only 1 unit of insulin to return her to normal blood glucose (90–100). But if she gets wildly out of control, say the high 200s or low 300s, it takes 2 units to get her back down to 200, plus a third unit to get her down to normal. She's lucky enough to be able to get back on track by injecting supplements of insulin, but as you point out, those Type 2s who don't take insulin just stay up there.

VIRGINIA: That's why we do the Fast Fast. It brings blood glucose down quickly. You become more sensitive to your own insulin and if you keep your blood glucose normal for a while, then you can often control it by watching your diet and you'll be less likely to have hunger attacks.

One reason why many Type 2s binge is the huge amount of insulin they're getting, especially when their blood glucose is out of control. As a Type 2 myself, I can "feel" an insulin rush during and after meals. It feels a little like the insulin reaction (blood glucose going too low) that Type 1s get when they overdose on insulin. When I'm getting an insulin surge I feel my lips quiver, but when I look in the mirror they aren't moving. Sometimes I get a little quivery feeling in my chest or neck. This is why many Type 2s will tell you that they aren't hungry all day—until they eat something. They get a rush of insulin with the food and that gives them the munchies. Then they proceed to eat all evening long. I'm sure that June can confirm this feeling. When you feel a surge of insulin in your body, it is very difficult not to eat something. I've found that if I can explain this reaction to people, they can live with it—and cope with it—better. For years they've probably been beating themselves up about having no willpower.

Besides these insulin surges that cause overeating, I feel that getting yourself into a "deprivation" mode can trigger the binge disorder;

at least it does for me. That's why the 20 percent fat diet works so well. The fact that you don't limit your serving sizes on the good-for-you foods gives you the strength to avoid the bad stuff. We have a patient with Type 2, a woman of thirty-five who has lost 30 pounds in the last four months. The other day she told me, "I can live like this forever, because I know I can have what I want when it comes to fruit, pasta, and veggies." I'm confident that she's going to be able to avoid the pit-fall of the deprivation mode and binge eating.

CARBOHYDRATES

JUNE AND BARBARA: In the recommended diets, sugar has always been a no-no, until the recent ADA pronouncements, but starch is OK. Why is this? Aren't they both carbohydrates?

VIRGINIA: As it turns out, there's very little difference. The bio-chemist calls starch a complex carbohydrate because it is a long chain of glucose molecules, as opposed to simple sugars that are made up of only a few glucose molecules. Dietitian Beverly Spears uses a great visual demonstration for this concept. She has several strings of those great big pop beads babies play with, which she has the patient break apart. Guess what? The long chain breaks apart just as easily as the short chain. This is the reason that the "glycemic index" studies found that white starches and white sugar are not very different in the effect they have on blood sugar. The glycemic index is a tool to measure the relative effect that different foods have on blood glucose. Different glycemic index studies have shown that white rice, mashed potatoes, and sugar have a similar effect on blood glucose. Does that mean that the person with diabetes should not eat potatoes or white rice? No, what it means is that you shouldn't eat a big bowl of white rice or mashed potatoes for a meal. A study reported in the *Diabetes Educator* (the journal of the American Association of Diabetes Educators) found that orange juice and Coca-Cola affect blood glucose exactly the same. What that means is that you should eat the whole piece of fruit instead of drinking juices. (Yes, I mean "no sugar added" juices as well; Mother Nature has already added the sugar.)

The sum total of all this is that a little sugar is not necessarily a problem for the person with diabetes. You can have goodies such as low-sugar cookies (animal cookies, vanilla wafers, gingersnaps, etc.), low-sugar cakes with no icing (Cool Whip makes a great cake or cupcake topping), or low-sugar frozen yogurt or ice cream.

GLYCEMIC INDEX

JUNE AND BARBARA: We might mention here, too, that the American Diabetes Association is definitely in accord. They say it's OK to have sugar if you limit yourself to no more than 10 percent of your total carbohydrate calories.

Getting back to the glycemic index, Table 4.1 shows that some complex carbohydrates are more complex than others and don't send blood sugar up as fast as mashed potatoes do. In this group are things like apples, sweet potatoes, black-eyed peas, and all kinds of beans. These are the "slow" carbohydrates, the ones that should help you keep your blood sugar more stable. Incidentally, Virginia, they're the very foods you've been telling us we should make the largest part of our meals—veggies and whole fruit.

TABLE 4.1   GLYCEMIC INDEX

This index compares the extent to which different carbohydrate foods raise blood sugar. Since glucose raises it the highest and fastest, it is assigned the index number of 100. The lower the number, the less impact the food has on raising blood glucose levels.

Simple Sugars		Fruits	
Fructose	20	Apples	39
Sucrose	59	Oranges	40
Honey	87	Orange Juice	46
Glucose	100	Bananas	62
		Raisins	64

continued on next page

TABLE 4.1   **GLYCEMIC INDEX** *continued*

Starchy Vegetables

Sweet Potatoes	48
Yams	51
Beets	64
White Potatoes	70
Instant Potatoes	80
Carrots	92
Parsnips	97

Dairy Products

Skim Milk	32
Whole Milk	34
Ice Cream	36
Yogurt	36

Legumes

Soybeans	15
Lentils	29
Kidney Beans	29
Black-eyed Peas	33
Garbanzos	36
Lima Beans	36
Baked Beans	40
Frozen Peas	51

Pasta, Corn, Rice, Bread

Whole-wheat Pasta	42
White Pasta	50
Sweet Corn	59
Brown Rice	66
White Bread	69
Whole-wheat Bread	72
White Rice	72

Breakfast Cereals

Oatmeal	49
All-Bran	51
Swiss Muesli	66
Shredded Wheat	67
Cornflakes	80

Miscellaneous

Peanuts	13
Sausages	28
Fish Sticks	38
Tomato Soup	38
Sponge Cake	46
Potato Chips	51
Mars Bars	68

The big problem we've always found with the glycemic index is that it only analyzes a small selection of carbohydrate foods and that leaves the majority of carbohydrates out there in mystery-land. That's why many dietitians say you have to test out individual carbohydrates on yourself and see which ones cause you to have normal or abnormal blood sugar. In other words, you create your own glycemic index by checking your blood sugar level after eating a portion of a particular carbohydrate food. That way you can learn to predict the potential effect of foods on blood glucose and plan accordingly.

VIRGINIA: That reminds me that the glycemic index rates pasta as a good carbohydrate. I've had some patients say they can eat a lot of pasta and not have a problem, but others say it really raises their blood glucose. I think I know the answer. The more you cook your pasta, the more you make it quickly digestible. Boiling too long changes the starch of pasta to sugar. So you need to cook it *al dente* in the true Italian manner and keep the portion small, such as 1 cup.

JUNE AND BARBARA: That's the way it tastes best, anyway. Now we need to know how long it takes different foods—protein and fat, as well as carbohydrate—to cause a rise in blood sugar.

VIRGINIA: Carbohydrate foods will cause a blood glucose peak about an hour after a meal. Only about 10 to 30 percent of the calories from protein convert to glucose, and they're released into the bloodstream over a period of four to eight hours after a meal. Fats may or may not cause a blood glucose rise. In some Type 2s, they don't tend to cause an increase in glucose, but in other Type 2s, where the body doesn't use glucose very well, the cells tend to use fat as a fuel source more easily, and therefore the glucose from the meal tends to be increased in the bloodstream because it is not being used by muscle cells (our old friend insulin resistance is at work here).

What you need to do to get a reasonable rise in glucose after a meal is to eat a *balanced* meal—carbohydrate plus some protein plus some fat (less than 30 percent of calories in fat). Considering the above peaking schedule for different kinds of nutrients, we can get a good postmeal level if we add lots of fiber besides the protein and the fat. Don't get me wrong about protein. I'm not suggesting a high-protein diet. In fact, a low-protein diet is better for all of us.

You can plan on 1 ounce of protein at breakfast, 1 or 2 ounces at lunch, and 3 ounces at dinner. This is a fairly low-protein diet, but by including a little protein with each meal, lots of vegetables both raw and cooked, and starches with fiber (brown rice, baked potato with skin), you get a better after-meal glucose; Type 2s get improved utilization of glucose by increasing insulin sensitivity.

JUNE AND BARBARA: We've heard that when you're trying to lose weight, it's not a good idea to drink your calories. Liquids slip down too easily, and since you don't get any chewing satisfaction from them, you may feel hungry and go off and eat a lot more calories in some more substantial form.

VIRGINIA: Yes, it's my philosophy never to drink calories. You can have so many good things like all those diet soft drinks that are calorie free, so why waste your calories on liquids? Also, liquid sugar absorbs so fast that you can't even cover it with insulin to get a decent blood sugar reading. We tell our patients to avoid all fruit juices and eat the fruit instead. Did you know that you have to smash eight apples to get just a half cup of juice, and then you've thrown away the best part—the fiber?

For people who are addicted to their juice in the morning, we suggest Crystal Lite's citrus blend flavor. It tastes like orange-pineapple juice and it has no calories. My personal favorite flavor is the pink grapefruit.

JUNE AND BARBARA: How do you feel about getting liquid calories via alcohol? We don't want to be accused of advocating drinking, but we feel it's our duty to acknowledge the big media blitz about the "French Paradox" of two glasses of red wine a day lowering cardiovascular risk and increasing HDL ("good" cholesterol). Not long after that revelation, we read in *Diabetes Care* (April 1992) about a new study from Bordeaux, France, which showed that two glasses of wine with a meal have no adverse effect on glycemic control in people with diabetes. In fact, there was a slower rise in glucose after the meal in non–insulin-dependent Type 2s than if they had water with their meal instead of wine. So you'd better hurry up and tell us what's wrong with drinking before the French lead us down the wrong path.

VIRGINIA: A "lite" beer or glass of dry wine with a meal is no big deal, but if you do serious drinking, you'll probably find that it does serious damage to blood sugar control. You should never drink alcohol on an empty stomach because your liver gets preoccupied with the alcohol and forgets to put glucose back into the blood when your blood sugar starts getting low. That's why people on pills or insulin are always advised to have their drink with a snack or meal.

It's important to remember, though, that there are 7 calories per gram of alcohol, just 2 calories less than fat! A 3-ounce glass of dry wine has 70 calories. If weight is a problem, you need to take that into consideration before you start following the French Paradox prescription. And, of course, with hard liquor you should use only sugar-free mixes. Better still, use sugar-free mixes without the alcohol!

JUNE AND BARBARA: We've often heard from dietitians that Type 1s need to count carbohydrates and Type 2s need to count calories. Is that true?

VIRGINIA: Yes, in fact we teach people who are learning to use Humalog or Regular insulin to count carbohydrates so they'll know how much insulin they need to take to balance their blood sugar. As I said before, we use a formula of 1 unit of Humalog or Regular insulin for each 10 to 15 grams of carbohydrate in order to get a good after-meal blood sugar. But it is important for each individual to test about an hour after a meal so that they can determine their own insulin-to-carbohydrate formula.

JUNE AND BARBARA: What about the so-called dietetic and diabetic foods? Of late we've noticed that there are mail-order food companies that handle nothing but special sugar-free sweets and treats for diabetics. Are they good for you and worth the usually inflated prices?

VIRGINIA: These candies, cookies, jams, and other items are usually made without sugar or their main enticement is that they're low calorie. I've heard dietitian Beverly Spears' talk on these a number of times. She gives a lesson in label reading. When the label says "no sugar added" and you look at how the product is sweetened, it may be with concentrated fruit juice, or with something like corn syrup, which is not sugar but has the same effect on blood glucose. The number of calories will often be no different from regular food. We often see this in cookies, especially. Dietetic cookies may have 30 calories apiece, just like regular cookies and at twice the price. We recommend eating regular cookies that are low in fat and sugar, such as gingersnaps, vanilla wafers, animal cookies, or plain little shortbread cookies. Read the labels. Find a cookie that has less than 2 grams of fat for each serving (which may be from two to six cookies, depending on the size). These are going to be much lower in price than dietetic varieties and cause little or no rise in blood sugar.

The other group of foods to watch out for are the dietetic candies. Most times these are sweetened with sorbitol, mannitol, or other substances with "ol" on the end. They all have a laxativelike effect. Hard candies or chocolates with mannitol or sorbitol as their sweetener will have fewer calories than regular sugar candies, because they are a little lower in fat. It's not the sugar that makes the difference, because sorbitol and mannitol sweeteners have about the same number of calories as sugar. But for some people, a very little bit of this type of product causes severe gas cramps and possibly diarrhea. (The last thing you want to do on a long trip is give your child a pack of Velamints with sorbitol.) Sometimes caramel corn or other specialty products advertised for diabetics are also sorbitol sweetened. These "dietetic" products cost more, and we don't think they're worth it. We like to teach the person with diabetes to have a little bit of sweets containing a little bit of sugar. A little bit of sugar is no problem in a well-balanced diet. Shop in regular markets and buy regular foods, not what's in the special sections of dietetic foods.

One of the interesting tidbits Beverly Spears discovered is that good old New York-style cheesecake does not cause much of a glycemic rise. That's because it's all fat and very little sugar. Some of us can't tolerate the calories of eating cheesecake very often, but for those who don't have a weight problem and especially for pregnant gals, this is a great alternative to eating cake. For Thanksgiving they can have pumpkin cheesecake. For the baby shower or other special occasion, they can have a small piece of cheesecake and feel like they're having a really yummy dessert without raising their blood sugar much.

FIBER

JUNE AND BARBARA: You've mentioned that fiber can slow down the rise in blood glucose after a meal. Dr. James Anderson, author of *Diabetes: A Practical New Guide to Healthy Living,* has long advocated a diet high in complex carbohydrate and fiber (HCF diet) for people with Type 2 diabetes. His maintenance diet for overweight diabetics calls for 50 grams of fiber a day for a 2,000-calorie plan. The American Diabetes Association recommends that the diet include up to 40 grams of fiber a day. Since most people when diagnosed with diabetes are probably eating only 10 or 11 grams of fiber a day, they're missing the benefits fiber can give them. And it's not all that easy to up the fiber in your diet.

VIRGINIA: To give you an idea of how difficult it is to get 50 grams of fiber, a serving of Grape Nuts (1/4 cup) has 3 grams of fiber, a serving of Cheerios has only 3 grams, and a serving of Rice Krispies has *no* fiber. You have to eat lots of vegetables, fruits, and beans to get 50 grams of fiber in your diet.

JUNE AND BARBARA: Table 4.2 shows some of the foods that are particularly high in fiber. By including some of these foods in your meals you can start building up to your 30, 40, or 50 grams a day.

TABLE 4.2   HIGH-FIBER FOOD CHART

(Listed in Descending Order of Fiber Content)

	Serving Portion	Grams of Fiber
Beans and Peas		
Black-eyed peas	1/2 cup	12.4
Kidney beans, canned	1/2 cup	7.9
Pinto beans	1/2 cup	5.3
Split peas	1/2 cup	5.1
White beans	1/2 cup	5.0
Breads and Crackers		
Pumpernickel	1 slice	3.8
Triscuits	6	3.3
Wonder high-fiber wheat or white	1 slice	2.9
Cornbread, whole-ground	1 piece (78 grams)	2.7
Graham crackers (2 1/2" square)	3	2.1
Cereals		
All Bran with extra fiber (Kellogg)	1/2 cup	14.0
Fiber One (General Mills)	1/2 cup	13.0
Raisin Bran (Post)	2/3 cup	6.0
40% Bran Flakes (Kellogg)	1/2 cup	5.0
Fruits		
Raspberries, fresh	1 cup	9.1
Blackberries, fresh	3/4 cup	6.7
Pear, fresh	1	5.0
Strawberries, fresh	1 1/4 cups	4.1
Prunes, dried	3 medium	4.0
Apricots, raw, with skin	4	3.5
Nectarine with skin	1	3.3
Orange, fresh	1	2.9
Apple with skin	1 small	2.8
Plums, fresh	2 medium	2.4

HIGH-FIBER FOOD CHART *continued*

	Serving Portion	Grams of Fiber
Grains		
Spaghetti, whole-wheat, cooked	1/2 cup	2.7
Rice, brown, cooked	1/2 cup	2.4
Popcorn, air-popped	3 cups	2.0
Vegetables		
Artichoke, cooked	1/2	7.6
Squash, winter, cooked	1/2 cup	3.6
Pumpkin, canned	3/4 cup	3.3
Asparagus, cooked	3/4 cup	3.1
Green beans, cooked	1/2 cup	2.8
Zucchini, cooked	1/2 cup	2.7
Broccoli, cooked	1/2 cup	2.4
Carrots, raw	1 medium	2.3

JUNE AND BARBARA: Try as you may, though, sometimes it just isn't possible to get up to that 50-gram level, especially if you eat a lot of meals out. We agree with dietitians who maintain that the very best way to get your fiber, as well as all your vitamins and minerals, is from the food you eat. We used to take a fiber supplement, but in recent years, we've tried to get our fiber from foods. Two good fiber sources that we plug into every day are Bran-a-Crisp, a high-fiber, low-carbohydrate crisp bread with 3.5 grams of fiber and La Tortilla Factory Low Fat Tortillas, which are made with 100 percent whole wheat flour, are 99 percent fat free, and each contains a whopping 9 grams of fiber. Plus, they're delicious. If you have trouble finding these in your market or health food store, contact us at 5623 Matilija Ave., Van Nuys, CA 91401 for a *Diabetic Reader* that tells how to get them.

VIRGINIA: High fiber in the diet has lots of advantages. Not only does fiber slow down the rise in blood glucose after meals, but it improves carbohydrate metabolism and lowers cholesterol and triglycerides. As if that weren't enough, fiber may also contribute to lower blood pressure and it can enhance weight loss in fluffy people.

You should eat a wide range of foods to include both kinds of fiber: soluble, such as oats, legumes, and fruits; and insoluble, such as wheat products and bran. High-fiber foods are low in fat and are very filling. If you get filled up on these good foods, you're less hungry and won't be tempted by a stray candy bar. The person who decides to try the high-fiber route must build up to it gradually and also increase fluids in the diet dramatically. High-fiber diets have social consequences, as a diet high in fiber will cause gas.

As for fiber supplements, they appear to provide benefit only if your diet is comprised of at least 50 percent of calories as carbohydrate.

JUNE AND BARBARA: What about dietary supplements of other kinds for Type 2 diabetes? Magazines and newspapers are always coming up with minerals and vitamins and even herbs that they claim will improve or even cure diabetes.

VIRGINIA: People with Type 2 diabetes should probably add a mineral supplement to their regimen that includes magnesium and chromium picolinate, as these have been found to increase insulin sensitivity in many people. Another supplement to add is vitamin E. Vitamin E has recently been found to improve your lipid levels and decrease the risk of heart attack. Also, ask your doctor about taking a small dose of aspirin daily to reduce the risk of heart disease. These are simple but really important areas to watch because cardiovascular disease is the major cause of death for us Type 2s.

SNACKING

JUNE AND BARBARA: Since we like people with diabetes to have as much flexibility as possible in their lives, how about skipping meals if the circumstances—such as plane delays in travel—might make it hard to come up with the right food at the right time?

VIRGINIA: Yes, you can skip meals as long as you're not on insulin. If you take one of the oral agents, you might start feeling a little low if you don't eat. Usually you won't, though, because your body makes extra insulin only in response to meals. If you don't have a meal for it to respond to, it won't make the insulin.

While skipping a meal once in a while is possible, it's really not a great idea because you may get too hungry and overeat at the next meal. Our dietitians strongly advise our patients always to get up and have a nice high-fiber cereal breakfast even if they feel like sleeping in and skipping that meal. Then have lunch. If you get hungry midafternoon, have a snack, something like fat-free yogurt—fruit yogurt that is sweetened with Nutrasweet tastes great and is under 100 calories. Low-fat cottage cheese makes a good snack, as do raw vegetables with low-fat ranch dressing. And, of course, fruit is the all-time great snack. They also strongly advise another snack at bed-time. The reason for all these meals and snacks is that by spreading your calories throughout the day, you're less likely to store as many of them as you do when you eat them all at once.

Let's say your total daily calorie intake is 1,800–2,000 calories. If you divide them into more frequent, smaller amounts, you'll be much more likely to use them as energy sources. If, on the other hand, you don't eat all day and then consume 2,000 calories at one meal, obviously your body can't make use of all that and actually stores a higher percentage of the calories.

JUNE AND BARBARA: We always recommend that you eat like a cat, not like a dog. The difference between the dining habits of these two favorite animal companions was brought home to us once when we were going to be out of town and wanted to leave some food for a neighborhood cat who always made it a habit to drop by for dinner—and sometimes breakfast and lunch! We got one of those cylindrical containers that you can fill up and as the cat eats, the food drops down into the feeding bowl. The feeder had a stern warning that it was to be used only for cats, never for dogs; if you used it with a dog, death might result! We asked the pet shop clerk why death would result if a dog used it. Was it that he might get his head stuck in the container and suffocate? No. The problem with dogs is they don't know when to stop. If you put a whole container of food out, the dog will dive in and, as the clerk said, "eat himself into oblivion." A cat, on the other hand, will just take a few mouthfuls of food now and then throughout the day—and sometimes throughout the night. Seldom if ever do cats eat large quantities at once, dog style. This is why, although there are such things as fat cats, you see them much more seldom than you do fat dogs. Dog owners often have to put their pets on diets because with the dog's typical one-big-meal-a-day program, they store up too much fat.

VIRGINIA: Yes, fat storage can be a hazard for all creatures great and small. But for a Type 2 it's a big-time hazard. That's because what we're talking about is building more fat, and more fat means more insulin resistance, and more insulin resistance just compounds our problems.

You may say, "Yes, but I'm not hungry until I eat. Then after the first few bites, I almost go crazy with hunger and it's a struggle not to overeat. I don't want to go through that more times a day than I already do."

I understand that terrible hunger feeling from experience. It's part of the disease. Food gives you a big insulin surge that makes you ravenous. From my experience, though, I also know that if you spread your food over the day and eat something every three or four hours, you'll find that you're far more able to control your eating and maintain your weight than if you eat all of your day's calories at one gigantic meal.

RIDING THE RADICAL RAPIDS:
THE LOW-CARBOHYDRATE, HIGH-PROTEIN DIET

JUNE AND BARBARA: Now we're going to present the minority opinion we mentioned earlier in this chapter.

The low-carbohydrate, high-protein diet is controversial to say the least. In fact, many health professionals find it upsetting because it calls into question everything they've believed—and taught patients—over the years. When we began discussing this diet in the *Diabetic Reader*, one dietitian wrote to cancel her subscription. Her doctor had forbidden her to read it because it raised her blood pressure so much—not *following* the diet, just *reading* about it.

But before we get totally emersed in the low-carbohydrate diet, let's talk about a much less controversial subject, carbohydrate counting. Keeping track of the exact amount of carbohydrate you eat at each meal is now being taught by many dietitians as a better way to manage diabetes. Why is carbohydrate counting so important? In her excellent audiotape *Carbohydrate Counting* (see Recommended Listening), dietitian Betty Brackenridge explains that some foods have a much greater effect on your blood sugar than others. And the big factor is carbohydrate. Ninety percent of the digestible carbohydrate you eat ends up as blood sugar. Carbohydrate comes in the form of starches, which you get from foods like potatoes, bread, pasta, and beans and from sugars, which you get from foods like fruit, milk, candy, and table sugar. Protein, which comes from meat, fish, poultry, beans, dairy products, and fats (which you seem to get from just about everywhere these days but especially from butter, margarine, salad dressing, and fried foods), yields small proportions of glucose. The glucose that comes from protein and fat tends to appear in the blood sugar gradually, up to several hours after the meal, while the sugars from carbohydrate shows up relatively soon after eating. So the amount of insulin needed to control your blood sugar after eating is closely related to how much carbohydrate you eat. This is true whether you take injected insulin or whether you depend on your body's own supply. What this means is that most people (maybe you're one of them) can do an excellent job of managing food intake for better blood sugar control by simply counting the grams of carbohydrate contained in the food they eat.

In the *Carbohydrate Counting Cookbook* (see Recommended

Reading), authors Tami Ross, R.D., C.D.E., and Patti Geil, R.D., C.D.E., point out, "The importance of counting carbohydrate has been apparent for some time. In 1935 the famed diabetes physician Elliott P. Joslin said, 'In teaching patients their diet, I lay emphasis first on carbohydrate values, and teach to a few only the values of protein and fat.'"

Do you agree with the benefits of carbohydrate counting?

VIRGINIA: Yes, I like the idea of helping people with diabetes understand the impact of carbohydrate counting and to a certain extent I do it myself. I also like the system devised by my friend and diabetes educator, Sue Perry in Santa Fe, New Mexico. In this plan the Type 2 patient is given a "budget" of the number of carbohydrate servings for each meal. The patient then uses after-meal blood sugar testing to fine-tune the budget. You might discover what your budget should be by starting very low with the Fast Fast (discussed at the beginning of this chapter) and then gradually keep adding carbohydrate until you see your blood sugar control start to slip away. Using that carbohydrate level as the limit of your budget, you can go from there. But as the authors of the *Carbohydrate Counting Cookbook* suggest, "Keep in mind that your tolerance for carbohydrate may change over time, so your carbohydrate goal . . . [is] not set in stone. Factors such as exercise, medications, pregnancy, weight gain, and physical activity can alter your carbohydrate requirements." So, I might add, can stress.

JUNE AND BARBARA: One of the nicest features of carbohydrate counting is that it's so easy. You only have to think of one dietary element. Food manufacturers are now required to include carbohydrates in the nutrition facts label. And, since you only have to count "effective carbohydrate"—the carbohydrate that affects your blood sugar—you can deduct the amount of fiber in a product from the carbohydrate. That lets you slip in a little more carbohydrate, which is always welcome. Several books to help you count your carbohydrates are available, including *The Carbohydrate Addict's Gram*

Counter by Richard F. Heller, Ph.D., and Rachael F. Heller, Ph.D., and *Carbohydrate, Calories, and Fat in Your Food* by Art Ulene, M.D. If you decide that this way of eating is a lifetime plan for you and you want to be more meticulous about it, a good accurate gram scale to find the number of grams in a specific food item would be of value. For example, if you look up an apple in a carbohydrate reference book, you'll find it has 13 percent carbohydrate. If you weigh it on a gram scale and multiply the weight by .13, *voilà*, you have the number of grams you'll be eating. We use the percentage chart in the *Pocket Pancreas* by John Walsh, C.D.E., and Ruth Roberts, M.A.

When people start playing the carbohydrate counting game and seeing the effect carbohydrate has on their blood sugars, they start thinking about a lower-carbohydrate diet, which, in turn, tends to lead them toward *the* low-carbohydrate diet. In fact, some people who read the first edition of this book achieved such excellent results with your Fast Fast that they wrote to us asking if there would be any problem with following the low-carbohydrate diet principle. We take it you don't go for this plan, because in your Fast Fast, you start adding back carbohydrate just as soon as blood sugars go down to normal.

VIRGINIA: I'll tell you why we don't recommend that you follow this kind of an extremely low-carbohydrate diet permanently. It hearkens back to the old Atkins weight-loss diet or the so-called drinking man's diet of the 1960s. It was discovered that if someone consumes less than 60 grams of carbohydrate a day, they go into a state of ketosis. That means they're burning their own body fat to convert it to fuel. Of course , they lose weight. The problem is that they're eating gigantic hunks of meat, as much as they want, and that increases their health risks. It increases some of the same risks that diabetes alone does.

A low- or no-carbohydrate/high-protein diet is dangerous on a long-range basis because it is by default a high-fat diet. Protein and fat hang out together. They're inseparable buddies. With a high-fat diet you can get very high blood cholesterol and very high low-density

lipoprotein levels, and both of these contribute to cardiovascular disease. Yet another risk with protein is that it's hard on the kidneys.
Actually, any diet that eliminates major food groups is not a good
lifetime solution.

We do not recommend that you adopt a diet that is extremely
low in carbohydrate and low in calories for more than a few days, just
long enough to get your blood sugars down. Some people can do a
Fast Fast to control blood sugars. They feel real good and have lots of
energy. I, on the other hand, will get a high level of ketones and am
liable to go out and attack a wheat field. Many people don't tolerate
it any better than I do. And, ketones make your breath smell funny.

JUNE AND BARBARA: Those are very logical reasons to be negative
about the diet. But we're glad you didn't perpetuate the mythical fear
many people hold that the ketones Type 2 diabetics develop on a
low-carbohydrate diet would lead to diabetic coma. Both Dr. Calvin
Ezrin (author of *The Type II Diabetes Diet Book*) and Drs. Michael and
Mary Dan Eades (authors of *Protein Power*) point out in their books
(see Recommended Reading) that the risk of diabetic coma is only
true for out-of-control Type 1s in ketoacidosis. The "mild, beneficial"
ketosis of the weight-loss phase of low-carbohydrate diets is a normal
stage of fat breakdown.

This brings us to the basic theory behind the low-carbohydrate
diet for weight loss. Exponents of the low-carbohydrate diet believe
that excess carbohydrate rather than fat causes weight gain in some
people because it stimulates the production and release of insulin
and insulin is a potent fat-building hormone. Indeed, the trend
toward more support for this alternative diet is gradually building
up. Dr. Julian Whitaker, long a passionate proponent of the high-
carbohydrate diet in his book *Reversing Diabetes*, in his January 1998
Health and Healing Newsletter reversed his "dogma" with this statement: "While I maintain my stance on the deleterious effects of
excessive fats, new research has convinced me that excessive carbohydrates pose similar risks."

A doctor on the Internet's LC Diabetes List avowed that

"Most M.D.s aren't up to speed on low carbohydrate, but because it is a radically different theory from current dogma, some inertia is to be expected." He said that you can find doctors who believe in low-carbohydrate diets and more and more are realizing "the inadequacies of the old paradigms." And more surprising, Alex Hass, author of *Everyday Low Carb Cookery*, said he understood low carbohydrate was being taught to some extent at Harvard Medical School. He added, "Unfortunately there will be many folks who acquire Type 2 diabetes and heart problems that could have been prevented had the word gotten out sooner."

Incidentally, Dr. Ezrin in his *Type II Diabetes Diet Book* manages to combine the best of both worlds. His is a low-carbohydrate diet that also controls fat intake, and his maintenance diet has more carbohydrate than many other low-carb diets. Since he's been in diabetes all his professional life—he trained at the University of Toronto, home of the discovery of insulin—he recognizes the fact that all people with diabetes are not created equal. Different folks have different carbohydrate needs and capacities, and the challenge is to find what your carbohydrate "budget" is.

We also want to confess that we have both been on a rather stringent low-carbohydrate diet for three years. June went on it because she was having trouble controlling her blood sugars when her insulin of choice, Pork Ultralente, was taken off the market. At about the same time Barbara, who had put on close to 10 pounds after a two-week pasta, pizza, and polenta festival of eating in Italy, decided she had to Do Something. That something turned out to be the low-carbohydrate diet. We basically followed Dr. Richard Bernstein's edict of 30 grams of carbohydrate a day. He divides it into 6 for breakfast, 12 for lunch, and 12 for dinner. He advises fewer carbohydrates at breakfast because so many diabetics find it the hardest meal of the day to keep their blood sugar normal. Following this plan, we tried to eat about the same amount of protein—enough to make you feel comfortable but not full—at each meal. And, we must confess, we just let the fats fall where they may. So far the diet has accomplished what we both wanted it to: June got her control back and

Barbara got rid of her weight. (However, it will return as inevitably as the swallows to Capistrano if she goes to New York and can't resist the wonderful breads or to Italy, where she can't resist the you-know-what.) The best part is that it hasn't harmed our cholesterol and triglycerides. Dr. Bernstein maintains that if your blood lipids (those two things we just mentioned) are normal—as ours were—prior to going onto the diet, they will stay normal. If they are high, they usually go down.

We describe our adventures on this diet in a 10,000-word special supplement in the 1998 edition of *The Diabetic's Book: All Your Questions Answered* (see Recommended Reading). And, we describe who has no business going onto it.

Despite our success on this diet, we are by no means recommending it to everyone. The mainstream high-carbohydrate, low-fat diet is much easier to follow in the sense that it fits better into the standard American (and Italian!) way of eating. Let's face it, any diet that virtually eliminates breads, rice, potatoes, pasta, pizza, corn, chips, and cereals rather cuts into the dietary staples everyone else is wolfing down. The mainstream diet will also make you feel more comfortable in dealing with diabetes health care professionals, since they almost uniformly condemn the low-carbohydrate diet as being unhealthy, and they generally won't support you in your desire to try it. So, you *will* need professional support. This is also not something you should try on your own, especially since, if you take insulin or certain pills, it may cause precipitous drops in your blood sugar and you may have some special condition (kidney damage or gout) that contraindicates this sort of diet.

However, this diet may be a life preserver and complication preventer for you if you've honestly, sincerely, and conscientiously tried to follow the mainstream high-carbohydrate, low-fat diet and have failed miserably at it—both your weight and your blood sugars have remained high. You may have even been accused of "cheating" (that dreadful word) by those health professionals who should know better. You may have reached the conclusion that diabetes is impossible and you're never going to be able to lose weight and achieve normal blood sugar so you might just as well give up and go eat a piece of pecan pie à la mode. This diet may give you another chance at success. That's why we call it "the diet of last resort."

We've received letters from diabetics who were furious. Their anger was not because, like the dietitian who canceled her subscription to the *Diabetic Reader*, they considered the diet outrageous and unhealthy. No, they were furious because "This is the only thing that's ever worked for me. Why has no one told me about it before? It must be some kind of conspiracy!"—which is why we insisted on telling you about it, controversial though it may be. It gives you another option in this disease of many options. Sorting through them and discovering the ones that work for you gives you infinite possibilities for success.

P.S. Internet surfers: If you want to learn more about the low-carbohydrate diet from people who are actually Doing It, you might join the LC-Diabetes. This is a support list for all persons controlling intake of carbohydrates as a method to manage diabetes and avoid diabetic complications. The purpose of the list is to share experiences, offer each other support, and chat about daily challenges in the spirit of sharing knowledge on the dietary and health issues of this diet. You should be warned, however, that information obtained here might not be accurate or medically appropriate for everyone. If you want to check it out, send e-mail to listserv@maelstrom. stjohns.edu with the message: sub lc-diabetes and your name.

VIRGINIA: We are not as far apart as you might think. I, too, have learned that controlling carbohydates is the answer to good control. I don't prefer to go a low as 30 grams a day, but I do feel that each of us has to find the balance in our diet that gives us good blood sugar control as well as feeling satisfied all day and not consumed with hunger by constantly thinking about what to eat next. Everyone should try to determine their own carbohydrate budget. Most people will find that eating vegetables (green beans, broccoli, squash, not corn or peas) fills you up and doesn't raise your blood sugar. I think that the recommended 50 percent carbohydrate was never meant to be filled with starch. There is a vast difference between $1/2$ cup potatoes and $1/2$ cup brussels sprouts. In fact, if everyone ate lots of veggies, they would find their blood sugars are better and their cholesterol improved, and they would feel full from moderate-calorie meals. Here's to veggie power!

CHAPTER ❦ 5

EMOTIONAL ASPECTS OF DIABETES:

My Enemy/My Friend

We remember well the day of Wednesday, July 29, 1992, because that was the day we picked up Mary, our new Scottish-Fold kitten. That day was made even more memorable by a report we heard on National Public Radio's "Morning Edition." It was the story of Larry Trapp, the Lincoln, Nebraska, Ku Klux Klan Grand Dragon and head of Nebraska's American Nazi Party. Trapp lost both of his legs in 1988 because of diabetes complications.

From childhood, Trapp's life had been consumed by hatred of all those who were different from him; Jews and blacks were his favorite hate targets. So it was only natural that when Cantor Michael Weiser and his family moved into Lincoln, Larry began a harassment campaign, calling them at all hours to deliver anti-Semitic threats such as, "You're going to be sorry you ever moved here, Jew boy," and putting cards in their mailbox saying things like, "The KKK is watching you, scum."

Understandably disturbed, the Weisers contacted friends and the police for help whenever these harassments occurred. But after a while, Michael and his wife, Julie, started examining their own feelings. They realized that they were the victims of hatred, yes, but they had also become haters themselves. They hated Larry Trapp.

This realization caused Michael Weiser to come to the personal decision that he was going to change. He was going to practice the love, understanding, and forgiveness that he preached in his sermons at the temple. Cantor Weiser says that in Judaism, "The highest thing that a human being can do is to make an enemy into a friend." But he acknowledged that most of us never do that. As he explains, "We have an enemy so we either avoid that enemy or we fight with that enemy."

He decided that the only solution to the enmity he felt toward Larry Trapp was to become friends with him. To make that happen, he launched his own harassment campaign against Trapp—a friendship harassment campaign. He began leaving messages on Trapp's answering machine that tried to point him in the direction of love rather than hate.

One day when Cantor Weiser was making one of his regular friendship harassment calls, Trapp picked up the phone and started shouting at him to stop calling. Weiser ignored the shouting and said simply and kindly, "I know you're disabled. Would you like a ride to the grocery store?"

Trapp was quiet for a while and then said, "No, but I thank you for asking."

A few nights later Trapp called Cantor Weiser and told him that he needed to talk. The cantor and his wife immediately went to Trapp's house. He confessed to them how lonely he was, and the Weisers stayed and talked with him for over four hours. Trapp later said he had never met anyone who showed such love and caring as they did. At the end of their evening together, Trapp symbolically removed the two swastika rings he was wearing and handed them to the Weisers, saying he didn't need them anymore.

A few months later, Trapp converted to Judaism. When his health worsened—he was dying of kidney failure caused by the diabetes—Julie Weiser quit her job in order to nurse him full time. During the last months of his life, Trapp spent his time meeting with people who were willing to rethink their racism, showing them how his life had changed for the better with love and without hate.

This moving story illustrates the Judaic principle of making an enemy into a friend. This is a principle that we all can and should apply to our daily lives.

Think about your diabetes. It's only human nature to regard it as an enemy that threatens and torments you every moment of every day. But, instead of letting yourself be consumed by hatred, try to turn that enemy into a friend, a friend who teaches you valuable lessons that you might not be able to learn in any other way, a friend who constantly pressures you to make changes for the better in your life.

In an article in the *Los Angeles Times*, "Forever Set in Your Ways at 30?" health writer Shari Roan reported that studies show that by age thirty or thirty-five, your personality is pretty much set for the rest of your life. Major changes are difficult to achieve and unlikely. There is, however, an exception to this rule: "Catastrophic events, such as developing a serious illness or losing a loved one, can change people."

Ms. Roan cited the example of Mark, a rock band singer who lived a wild and dangerous life that included taking drugs. When a van in which Mark was riding crashed, he was left paralyzed from the waist down. Mark now considers this accident the best thing that ever happened to him. It spurred him to get off drugs, go to college and on to graduate school, and then to launch into a successful professional career. As he says, "I don't think I would be here today if this hadn't have happened."

In a study of people who had experienced significant events in their lives, either positive or negative, psychologist Richard G. Tedeschi at the University of North Carolina found that negative events are the ones most likely to cause people to make changes. "Negative life events are so affecting that they call into question a lot of the usual ways of operating that people have adopted. Only because they're so traumatic do they pull people off their usual path."

Dr. Tedeschi goes on to say that people who have been transformed by negative events "often adopt a different philosophy of life . . . they begin to feel that life is good and useful; they become more expressive, more empathetic and tolerant."

The strangest revelation of this study is that profound *positive* events don't change people dramatically. This is because positive events don't challenge our basic ideas about living and what life is all about the way negative events do. In other words, unlikely though it may seem to you at the moment, diabetes can improve your life more than winning the lottery! It can, that is, if you neither avoid it nor fight it but turn it into a friend.

We'll now ask Virginia to show you some of the emotional steps you can take to establish that friendship and make it a long-lasting one.

—*June and Barbara*

DENIAL

JUNE AND BARBARA: We all know that people have different emotional reactions to a diagnosis of diabetes. Some have a healthy fear of what might happen to them, so they go to work on this diabetes thing. They get medical advice—and take it! They read, they go to support groups, and they take charge of their own health. They may become healthier than they were before they ever heard of diabetes. This group, unfortunately, is by far the minority.

What most people do at first—and this is a common strategy of self-protection when we feel overwhelmed—is simply deny the diagnosis. We hear the word "denial" a lot in modern life. "He's in denial" means that in order to function at all, the person must push whatever has happened that he doesn't like so far back in his mind that he doesn't even recognize its existence. For those of you who aren't familiar with denial, maybe this parable will illustrate what it's like.

The Parable of Denial

Once there was a man named George who deeply resented the fact that there was such a thing as gravity and that his life was so affected by it. He detested gravity from the very moment he first became aware of it when he was five years old. He was holding his mother's favorite antique bud vase. It slipped from his fingers and fell and shattered on the floor. He never forgot how upset his mother was.

He loathed the fact that snow and rain and hail and apples and everything else dropped down, never up or sideways. He hated tripping and falling and banging his knees—all because of that #$@%^&* gravity. George began to spend most of his time brooding about gravity and how it loused up what would otherwise have been a perfectly lovely world.

As time passed, his resentment got worse. He despised gravity and the restrictions it imposed upon him more and more until he finally could stand it no longer. He decided he was just going to ignore its existence. "I'm not going to let this gravity thing ruin my life," he announced.

From that day forward George pretended gravity wasn't there. If he held a piece of china or crystal in his hand, he let go of it and ignored the fact that it fell and broke. Before long his entire set of china and crystal was destroyed. He dropped his dachshund puppy so often that it would no longer come to him when he called. In fact, the puppy would hide when he came into the room. Then, one day George was at work looking out the window of his office, which was on the twelfth floor. It was such a nice day that he decided he'd go for a stroll. He opened the window, stepped out, dropped twelve stories, and broke every bone in his body. He's now in traction in the hospital waiting for his bones to knit, with an elaborate pulley system holding up his limbs against the force of gravity.

The moral of this parable is that you can't change a situation with denial, and you'll only hurt yourself if you try.

Denial in reference to diabetes is a word we hear constantly from the lips of health professionals. So tell us, what is your secret of helping people overcome this formidable barrier to coping with and controlling diabetes?

VIRGINIA: I've just finished reading four Tony Hillerman books. They're wonderful stories about the Navajo people, and this question of denial reminds me of the Navajo word *horzo*. According to Hillerman, *horzo* is their term for being out of harmony. That's how I think most people feel when they experience the news that they have diabetes.

I rarely meet anyone who is totally surprised by the diagnosis. Usually they have had a suspicion, or else they have suspected they had something worse than diabetes. Nevertheless, when the diagnosis is confirmed there is almost always a period of grieving. The grief is often related to the losses that they anticipate diabetes will entail. Many times these are losses they have heard about or maybe seen in family members with diabetes: loss of freedom to eat what they want, loss of being able to schedule their time any way they feel like, loss of health or limbs or sight, even loss of life.

We approach each newly diagnosed person differently, depending on circumstances. For example, if the person is a pregnant lady, we cannot afford the time to work through the grief in a leisurely manner. We must get her blood glucose under control immediately. Because we're dealing with the health of her child, usually the patient can muster the spirit and energy to assist us with the task.

Many people, without the motivation of a pregnant woman, react with anger. They're angry at having diabetes and sometimes take it out on the health care practitioner who gives them the news—the old shoot-the-messenger strategy. Others simply won't accept the diagnosis. I've seen people go from doctor to doctor to doctor trying to get one of them to give a different diagnosis.

My approach is to support such people with care and information. I tell them that I have diabetes and have had it for eighteen years. This usually helps them see that there is life after diagnosis.

Then I try to give them information on how they will be able to live with diabetes day in and day out. I allow people to be unhappy about diabetes. Nobody has to like it, but we do have to go on living, and if you control your diabetes, you can live with it better and easier and healthier.

I encourage people to keep coming back for appointments at our diabetes center at least every two weeks until we see that they have a handle on the situation. We only work on survival skills for the first few months. People don't remember any of the complicated stuff if we try to teach it to them while they're still in a state of shock over the diagnosis. People look as if they're paying attention, and they may think they're on top of things, but if you ask them later what they remember about the first month or two after the diagnosis, often they can hardly remember a thing. This is true of many stressful events in people's lives. Can you remember the funeral of a close relative? Details of a divorce? We realize that the diabetes diagnosis is a traumatic event in their lives and try to give them only simple steps to follow.

How do I know this? When I was diagnosed with diabetes, I tried to approach it the way I do most things in my life—intellectually. "If I just find out everything about it, it won't affect me." Well, it affected me just like everyone else—with denial, grief, and depression. Because I know how they feel, I always try to encourage people to go easy on themselves for several months, to give themselves a chance to adjust to the diagnosis, and to learn that living with diabetes is not as bad as they thought it would be.

After they've mastered the survival skills of diabetes (how to test blood sugar, take medication, and follow a simple diet), then we can move into the advanced course. We know when they're ready for this because they start asking questions. We also realize that we may have to repeat some of the information about survival skills at this time, because they were in a diagnosis trance the first time we told them.

Then we start them on our "In Charge" course. This is an ongoing program where we give advanced lessons in living with diabetes:

for example, how to eat out, how to adjust medications, how to prevent complications.

At the conclusion of this course, most people are ready for scheduled visits to their doctor every three months plus checking in with diabetes educators from time to time for some fine-tuning. We find that many of our patients come in for a visit just to chat about how things are going and to find out if there is anything new in diabetes management technology that they need to know.

JUNE AND BARBARA: What do you do when you meet people with hard-core denial for whom your standard procedures don't work?

VIRGINIA: Yes, we sometimes meet people who can look at any evidence and only see what they want to see. For people like this, calling in family members or close friends may help. But sometimes we just have to wait them out and let them know how the disease is affecting them and give them plenty of space so that they can come back for help and still save face.

There's one young man we see in our practice that took us six months to get in for diabetes education. He was diagnosed with Type 2 diabetes although he's only thirty-six. He came to see one of our endocrinologists because his primary-care physician had sent him. He was a very busy business owner and was upset that these doctor visits took up so much time. His mother has diabetes and he knew exactly what to do without instruction—or so he thought. When he failed to keep his appointment with the Diabetes Network, we called and arranged a new one. He called and canceled. We arranged new appointments again and again. Again and again he canceled.

The way we finally got him to come in was by arranging the appointment with his wife, who realized the importance of good control. To make sure he got there, she came to the Center with him. Although it took many broken appointments to get him into the Center and out of denial and on track, he's finally getting into good control. His wife still comes with him to the appointments, and the two of them will be starting the "In Charge" class in two weeks.

MOTIVATION

JUNE AND BARBARA: Right up there with denial as a major emotional problem in diabetes is motivation: trying to make yourself do the things you know you should do for your diabetes and yourself. Usually denial is a one-time thing and once you get rid of it, it's gone forever. But that need to keep motivated is something you will always have to struggle with. Just how do you keep yourself motivated day after day, year after year, your whole life long?

VIRGINIA: That's a tough one! Almost every time I go to a diabetes conference for health professionals, there's a session on how to motivate your patients. The problem with diabetes is it's relentless. It's there day in and day out. It never goes away. It never lets up. If you get disgusted and decide that you'll just forget about it for a while, it will sneak up and whap you up the side of your head to remind you that it's still there.

ATTITUDE

JUNE AND BARBARA: Well, since it is always there and you do need to do all those day-in-and-day-out (boring!) things to take care of your disease, what can you do about making yourself keep on keeping on with it?

VIRGINIA: You need to get the right attitude about it. You probably think, "I'm sick and tired of fooling around with this diabetes thing every day. I'm sick and tired of never taking a break from it." And yet if I were to ask you, "Aren't you sick and tired of having to eat and drink every day? Do you pick up a piece of fruit or a glass of iced tea and say, 'I just hate it that I have to keep putting these things into my mouth and swallowing them every day for the rest of my life!'" No, you generally don't complain about that. You don't complain that you have to go to the bathroom several times a day forever or that you have to brush your teeth after each meal. There are a lot of things that we have to do all the time that we don't complain about. That's where that right attitude comes in. We have to decide that our diabetes routines are a basic part of life like taking baths and sleeping and breathing and do them without getting all worked up about it. That way, instead of being an odious chore, they become almost automatic and we can turn our thoughts to more pleasant things.

JUNE AND BARBARA: It also helps if, instead of grumbling and muttering about your odious chores and how deprived you feel and other disagreeable things, you focus on what's good about your life, the things that make you happy—in other words, develop more of an optimistic attitude.

VIRGINIA: That's my philosophy. I've always felt that taking a positive approach, seeing the glass as half full rather than half empty, seeing the doughnut rather than the hole, has been very important to my success in life.

But even though I'm generally very positive and optimistic, I have to admit there's one area in which I'm not. I'm a pessimist about optimism. That is to say, I'm not very optimistic that people who are very pessimistic will ever turn optimistic. In my experience people who see the glass as half empty and who only see the hole in the doughnut hardly ever change.

JUNE AND BARBARA: This reminds us of something we once read in an autobiographical novel by James Kirkwood, the author of *A Chorus Line*. The title of the novel, *There Must Be a Pony*, was from a story about twin boys. One was an incurable optimist; the other an incurable pessimist. Their father, who was trying to give each son a more balanced perspective on life, hit upon a scheme. On Christmas Eve he filled one room of the house with every toy and video game a boy could ever dream of having, and put a tag with the pessimist's name on the door. He filled another room from floor to ceiling with equine excrement and put the optimist's name on that door. The next morning he told the boys where to find their presents. An hour later he came back to see how each had reacted to his gift.

The pessimist was sitting on the floor in the midst of all his toys, sobbing and wailing and miserable because he couldn't decide which toy to play with first. The optimist was laughing and singing and whistling, merrily shoveling all the equine excrement.

"What's going on here?" asked the father. "Why are you so happy?"

"Gee, Dad," replied the son, "I figure that there must be a pony here somewhere."

Optimists we don't really want to change. It's the pessimists we'd like to do a little attitude adjustment with. Why do you figure it's so hard to get them to change?

VIRGINIA: Maybe it's because there's no motivation for them to change because they keep proving themselves right all the time, and that gives them a kind of perverse satisfaction. The militant pessimist will also tell you that he's never disappointed. He thinks of himself as a realist and regards those of us who are very positive and who see things optimistically as perfect fools.

But the thing about being optimistic and seeing things in life positively is that you often prove yourself right. When I look back on my life I see that almost everything has turned out positively. I am where I am because of how things evolved, and I am happy where I am. How can I—or anybody else—say I'm not in the right place?

Once when I was introducing myself to a class and telling them that I had Type 2 diabetes, a patient in the front row looked up at me and said, "Well, how do you like it so far?" And you know how you tell the truth when you're not really thinking about it? I looked at him and said, "Well, actually it's been a tremendous professional advantage." It's true. To me diabetes has been a positive experience in many ways.

JUNE AND BARBARA: To us, too! We wouldn't have had half the experiences we've enjoyed and met one-hundredth of the wonderful people we now know—including Virginia!—without diabetes. We know of many people for whom diabetes has had a positive impact— people who wouldn't have become doctors or nurses or dietitians or exercise therapists or psychologists if they hadn't had diabetes and been determined to learn more about their disease and to help others. We even know two young women who found the loves of their lives through diabetes. One was a diabetes teaching nurse who met her husband when he was the representative of one of the meter companies who was calling on her hospital. The other love story is a bit more complicated. The woman had diabetes and it inspired her brother to invent the Medicool, which keeps insulin cool when you travel, hike, drive in the car, etc., and even keeps it warm if you're off in the snow. (Come to think of it, this is a double diabetes positive— a successful business and true love!) At any rate, the woman and her brother had a booth at a medical trade show to demonstrate the Medicool. Working in the booth next to theirs was the president of a company making another medical product. Between exhibit hours, they all got to talking and the upshot is that she became engaged to the booth neighbor and now they're happily married.

We're so fascinated with how-diabetes-brought-me-happiness stories that we're collecting them. If you come up with such a positive tale, we hope you'll write to us and tell us about it. We'll publish it in *The Diabetic Reader* so everyone can have their spirits lifted. (Write to us at 5623 Matilija Ave., Van Nuys, CA 91401 to tell us your story or to request a *Diabetic Reader*.)

But it's not just people with diabetes who need to have a positive approach and a spirit of optimism. Their friends and family members need that attitude, too.

VIRGINIA: A good example of this is Cathy Feste, who is a diabetes educator as well as a person with diabetes. She tells the story about what happened when she was a child and was in the hospital just after being diagnosed. She asked her mother, "What does it mean that I have diabetes?"

Her mother said, "It means that our family will all learn to eat better and we will all be healthier." We should all be so lucky as to have family members who take that kind of approach. It really rubs off onto the person with diabetes. All diabetes educators are inspired by Cathy's positive approach to managing diabetes both for herself and for her patients.

But still it remains a challenge for diabetes educators to take a person who is very depressed or who sees diabetes as a tremendous burden and turn this attitude inside-out into a positive one. And it's an even greater challenge for the person him- or herself.

It's funny how life gives us gifts that we can use positively or negatively. It makes me think of my friend Marci Draheim from Cedar Rapids, Iowa. Marci is a wonderful diabetes educator who also is an accomplished musician. She writes and arranges her own music and uses the power of music to help people experience their emotions in a positive way. She expresses her feelings about helping people with diabetes with a beautiful ballad she composed, called "I'll Be Here for You." She is a perfect example of a person using the gifts God gave her to help others.

JUNE AND BARBARA: Is there any way to effect an attitude change in depressed and negative people and get them to start using their own natural gifts in a positive way?

VIRGINIA: It's no secret that helping other people is a key to helping yourself. I encourage my patients to get involved in the American Diabetes Association or the Juvenile Diabetes Foundation as volunteers. When you're working with other people and trying to help them, it's much more difficult to focus on how miserable you are yourself. So get involved, if not with diabetes, then with some other organization that interests you. Focus on doing something positive for other people. I guarantee it will drive a lot of the negative out of your own life.

Finally, I have to say to discouraged diabetics: Lighten up and don't be so serious about it. Maybe right now diabetes is on the front page of the newspaper of your life. It's not something that will ever get out of the news, but it can certainly be moved back to the lifestyle section or maybe even the comics page. It certainly doesn't need to be forever printed in bold front-page headlines like "BOMB EXPLODES!" or "WORLD COMES TO AN END!"

FAMILY AND FRIENDS

JUNE AND BARBARA: It's often said that diabetes is a family disease in the sense that it has an impact on the entire family, not just the person who has it. Just what goes on in families when diabetes raises its ugly head?

VIRGINIA: The way I put it is: People don't have diabetes; families have diabetes. Diabetes affects the entire family and may change the relationships and communication patterns among all family members. Family members may experience the same fears and anxieties as the person with diabetes—sometimes even more intensely. To add to that negative, the diabetic may feel as though he or she has a "low position" in the family and has no right to expect family support or assistance with diabetic routines or crises. Conversely, the diabetic may feel a role diminishment or power dilution if the rest of the family is handing out advice and instruction on his or her daily activities.

The situation grows even worse when the diabetic person decides to keep the disease private and not allow any family participation in order to protect the family from the stresses of diabetes. Or the person with diabetes may not allow the other members any involvement by simply ignoring the hazards of out-of-control diabetes and doing nothing much to manage it. If the family and the diabetic have an unspoken pact to ignore diabetes management, they become "coconspirators" in the diabetes denial racket. This is often displayed by the nondiabetic members encouraging the diabetic to go off the prescribed diet with tempting goodies or by planning activities that make it difficult or impossible to stay on the regimen. Diabetics will participate in this racket, because it's then possible for them to temporarily allay nagging thoughts about their inability to participate in activities like other people. It's as if they think they can avoid feeling the pain and fear of complications and possible loss of life. But in fact, diabetes cannot be ignored. Denial of fears and failure to communicate feelings just cause more stress and emotional pain for everyone concerned.

I can't emphasize too strongly the fact that enlisting your family members in active participation with diabetes management is the first step to good control.

JUNE AND BARBARA: That may not be easy to do. We've seen husbands and wives really irritated because one or the other has diabetes. Sometimes they resent diabetes and all the expense and trouble it can cause. One spouse can be extremely critical because the other cannot seem to handle diabetes well. Occasionally we've witnessed loud family arguments over aspects of diabetes, real knock-down-drag-outs in public. So how do you go about creating good, positive family involvement?

VIRGINIA: There are several important steps.

1. Give your family permission to participate in your diabetes management. This is the step most often neglected and the primary reason people don't receive support. Sharing your life together means sharing the difficulties as well as the joys. Invite other family members to participate in diabetes activities such as support groups, education classes, and diabetes association meetings. Remember that an invitation can be accepted or declined. Do not be judgmental about this.

2. Openly communicate your feelings. All members of the family must have the opportunity to express their fears and anxieties about diabetes, its complications, the restrictions of diabetes management, and especially their feelings about activities they may find repugnant, such as blood glucose monitoring or shots. Just getting people to openly express their feelings helps diminish the impact of those feelings.

3. Everyone in the family needs to learn the principles of diabetes management in order to give effective support. The whole family needs to get as much education about diabetes as possible. Each person needs a realistic understanding of what to expect from diabetes and what to do to ensure the best possible outcome.

4. You can make everything more comfortable for everyone, including yourself, by accepting diabetes rather than denying it. If you can't accept your diabetes, you'll find it difficult to accept support from others. Being in a position of dis-ease with diabetes leads to a constant feeling of not being OK, so your self-concept is diminished. Acknowledge that you're an OK person, a good person, and that diabetes is not a reflection of who you are. If you have a feeling of being at fault about having diabetes, this guilt and anguish will color all your relationships and interactions with others.

5. Listen to love! You should actively translate the comments and suggestions about your diabetes management made to you by your family members as expressions of love and caring. That's what they are. If your family didn't care about you, they wouldn't bother to comment on your diabetes activities at all. You can transform your relationships by reinterpreting what may have appeared to you as annoying criticisms into what such comments truly are: expressions of love and concern. This is what any psychologist will tell you, and I know it to be true.

STRESS

JUNE AND BARBARA: It's impossible, as you know, to talk about feelings and emotions without talking about stress. And stress, as any experienced diabetic knows, can play havoc with blood sugar. June was once stunned when she found out that facing a particularly worrisome situation caused her blood sugar to shoot up from around 100 to over 200 in less than fifteen minutes.

VIRGINIA: I could write an entire chapter on stress and diabetes, because it's such a knockout punch to blood sugar control.

JUNE AND BARBARA: Why don't you start out by defining stress so we'll all be perfectly clear on what it is?

VIRGINIA: Stress is any change in your environment that causes the body to activate its stress response and release stress hormones. These hormones are meant to rev up your energy so you can fight or run from the threat. This is the well-known "fight or flight" response to danger that is left over from primitive times when there were all those lions and tigers out there, not to mention lots of club-wielding two-footed enemies. What happens is the adrenal glands are alerted and they cause the release of glucagon (the opposite hormone from insulin; it raises blood sugar). Glucagon in turn signals the liver to release its stored glucose. This extra glucose is what causes the problem for us diabetics, because we can't make enough insulin to match the highly increased glucose levels. That's why June's blood sugar shot up like that. Her injected insulin wasn't enough to cover the extra glucose triggered by the unanticipated stressful event.

JUNE AND BARBARA: What kinds of events and emotions cause this "fight or flight" response?

VIRGINIA: Both physical stresses and emotional stresses activate the response. Illness, pain, infection, surgery, pregnancy—all these physical stresses raise blood glucose because of the release of stress hormones in the body. Probably more common in our daily lives, though, are the emotional stressors like work pressure, family problems, fights with your mate, money difficulties, hurricanes and earthquakes, and the endless upsets and crises people face in modern life.

JUNE AND BARBARA: Some people seem to be under *constant* stress because they have a lawsuit pending, or are in the midst of a divorce or child custody fight, or are trying to care for an elderly parent and take care of their children at the same time, and so on. We have found, too, that diabetes itself causes plenty of stress in most people's lives. Wouldn't you agree that diabetes is another constant stress?

VIRGINIA: I couldn't agree more. Ordinary events that aren't stressful for nondiabetics become major emergencies for the person with diabetes—things like, "Dinner will be late this evening," or "Your suitcase hasn't arrived with the rest of the plane's luggage." At any moment of the day you can find something that interferes with what you're supposed to be doing for your diabetes at that particular time. Tests showing high blood sugars can generate all kinds of fear: fear of blindness, kidney failure, or foot amputation. Not having the money to afford the test strips causes stress. I could go on and on. That's why at the Diabetes Network we teach our patients about the damaging effects of stress and how to change their response to it with stress management strategies.

JUNE AND BARBARA: Ever since we wised up about stress and its effects on health we've been working on ways to handle it. In fact, our *Diabetic's Total Health Book* is full of stress-reducing techniques, from exercise, meditation, and visualization to such far-out methods as pets, travel, laughter, and hugs. Let's hear your antistress ideas, Virginia, as life in the twenty-first century looks as if it's going to feature new and weird stresses that we've never encountered before. We all need to be acquainted with every form of stress therapy that's been invented—and then some.

VIRGINIA: I'm glad you realize you can't avoid stress, and therefore the more you practice the management strategies that work for you, the better. Here are my ideas on how to help yourself come to grips with stress:

Reduce the frequency of stressful incidents

1. Make changes in family, social, and work commitments. Find activities that provide pride of accomplishment and satisfaction.

2. Set attainable goals and reasonable expectations so that disappointments do not become major stress points.

3. If you take insulin, learn to adjust your diabetes regimen and lifestyle so that the likelihood of severe insulin reactions is lessened; always carry glucose tablets and snacks.

Reduce the intensity of the stress response

1. Learn Conscious Relaxation and practice it regularly (see the Conscious Relaxation exercise that follows).

2. Use meditation or prayer.

3. Decrease consumption of stimulants such as caffeine and nicotine.

Increase physical activity

1. Exercise reduces stress by relaxing muscle tension and increasing cardiovascular function.

Focus your energy

1. Identify the areas in your life that consistently result in frustration.

2. Control what can be controlled, and accept what can't be controlled. Remember, it's easier to ride a horse in the direction it's going.

3. Take action! Set your priorities. List tasks and break them into manageable sizes. Be realistic and flexible about time frames to achieve your goals.

Conscious Relaxation Exercise

Practice this exercise in a comfortable place with little likelihood of interruption. If you fall asleep doing the exercise, as some people do, plan for awakening, if you're doing this on a short time frame (such as a lunch break at work). Get into a comfortable seated or lying position without crossing your arms or legs. Read over the exercise and then do it for yourself, using a similar scenario, or read it onto a tape and play the tape back. You may want to put your favorite relaxing music on the tape as well. Similar types of relaxation exercises are available on commercially recorded tapes.

Start this exercise by taking a deep breath . . . and letting it out very slowly. Feel the tension going out with the air. Throughout your busy day, deep breathing can be a quick and effective relaxation exercise. Put a small dot of colored tape on your clock at work and let it be a reminder to you that every time you look at the clock you will take two deep breaths.

Take another deep breath and as you let the air out slowly, allow your eyelids to gently close. Feel your body settle into your chair and get very comfortable where you're sitting or lying. Now you will begin relaxing by talking to the muscles of your body and allowing them to get completely relaxed. Start at your head. Feel the muscles of your scalp getting very relaxed. Your head will begin to feel warm and relaxed and your forehead will relax. Notice that your face is relaxing and smoothing out as you feel the tension leaving your muscles. Notice the relaxed warm feeling moving around to the back of your head and neck and your head is feeling heavy and relaxed. Allow your head to sink deeper into your pillow or chair or to fall forward on your chest as your neck muscles lose all tension. Feel a warm flow of relaxation moving all around your neck into your shoulders and notice your shoulders drop as all effort leaves the muscles.

Now take another deep breath as you allow all tension to leave your head, neck, and shoulder area. Feel the wave of relaxation moving down your arms as all tension in the muscles of your upper arm, lower arm, and hands now flows out through your fingertips. Your arms are now completely relaxed and feel warm and heavy. Feel the warm, relaxed feeling moving across your chest and into your back. You can feel the tension leaving all the muscles of your back and abdomen as you sink deeper into your chair. Now allow that warm wave of relaxation to move through your lower back and buttocks and into your thighs. Feel a wave of relaxation moving into your legs as all tension leaves the muscles and flows through your knees, lower legs, and ankles. All tension and effort is now leaving your body through your toes, leaving the muscles completely relaxed and warm.

Now take another very deep breath and as the air flows out feel a final wave of warm relaxation wash over your body from head to toe, removing any tension left in any muscles. Now we will get into a deeper level of relaxation by counting down to the deepest level of relaxation. You will get more and more relaxed with each count as we count from 10 down to 1. You will hear the cue words "calm and relaxed" often. These will be your cues so that at any time, any place, you can return to this same level of relaxation by saying to yourself "calm and relaxed" and taking two deep breaths.

As we begin the count, imagine yourself on a beautiful, warm day with the sun shining in a blue sky. You are lying on a thick, fluffy cloud. You are completely supported, your body is totally comfortable and relaxed. Feel the gentle rocking of this beautiful white cloud as it gently floats you toward your most favorite spot on earth. Begin floating downward as we count 10 . . . calm and relaxed . . . 9 . . . you are floating gently toward your perfect place . . . 8 . . . calm and relaxed, deeper and deeper . . . 7 . . . feel the warmth and gentle rocking of your cloud . . . 6 . . . calm and relaxed . . . 5 . . . you are floating toward the place you most enjoy being, it can be a real place or a place you have only imagined . . . 4 . . . calm and relaxed . . . 3 . . . sinking deeper and deeper into relaxation . . . 2 . . . see your favorite spot . . . you are more relaxed than you have ever been . . . 1 . . . you are completely calm and relaxed . . . your cloud has brought you gently to your perfect place . . . look around . . . you can see in detail how beautiful this place is.

Look at yourself in this picture . . . notice how relaxed and healthy you look in your perfect spot . . . take a deep breath and say to yourself . . . "calm and relaxed" and know that you can return to this feeling of calmness and relaxation at any time by taking two deep breaths and saying to yourself "calm and relaxed."

Look at yourself in this picture and see yourself as healthy and happy and solving any problems you may have. You are now in a state of complete calm, health, and happiness. As you watch yourself in the picture you can see yourself getting healthier, handling all your day-to-day concerns with ease and grace. You can see that this feeling of relaxation will stay with you throughout your day. You will now leave your special place but your feeling of well-being and relaxation will stay with you and you will feel refreshed and full of energy. You will become more and more alert as we count from 1 to 4 and you will be fully awake, alert, and relaxed and feeling wonderful . . . 1 . . . 2 . . . 3 . . . 4 . . . welcome back.

SEX

JUNE AND BARBARA: Although this is as much a physiological issue as a psychological one, this might be as good a place as any to discuss sexual problems sometimes associated with diabetes since they can have such an emotional impact on all concerned. Breaking with tradition, let's put the gentlemen first. Does Type 2 diabetes cause impotence?

VIRGINIA: I hate to be the bearer of bad tidings, but yes, it can. Studies have reported that up to 50 percent of diabetic men over the age of fifty have some degree of impotence. In fact, after many other symptoms of diabetes have been ignored, impotence is sometimes the symptom that finally drives men to the doctor where they're first diagnosed as diabetic.

The primary physiological cause of this is neuropathy (nerve damage). The nerves that serve the penis and are responsible for erection become damaged by many, many years of high blood sugar. This causes an inability to achieve and maintain an erection. As with the other complications of diabetes, maintaining normal blood sugars can prevent this. Naturally, it's best to prevent it, since it is understandably very upsetting to a man. His libido is still intact, but he is unable to perform sexually. This can be extremely distressing not just for a man, but for the woman in his life as well.

JUNE AND BARBARA: What should a man do when confronted with impotence?

VIRGINIA: The first step is to have an evaluation by a urologist because there can be other reasons besides diabetic neuropathy for impotence and erection difficulties. If, after all the tests are done, the urologist ascertains that diabetes is the culprit and the problem is physiological, not psychological, there are some very good ways to help with this problem.

Among the best are the vacuum erection devices. With these, a tube is placed over the penis and air is removed to create a vacuum. The vacuum simply pulls blood into the penis and causes an erection. These devices are not very expensive, don't require surgery, and have been helpful to many couples. The cost is often covered by medical insurance, including Medicare.

Another system that some people have found effective is to use injections of a drug such as papaverine or phentolamine that will cause blood to be pulled into the penis and cause an erection.

Some people resolve the problem with surgical implants, either inflatable or semirigid. Although some men and their wives have found these to be very effective, some serious complaints have been reported about them. Sometimes additional surgery has been required to replace defective implants, to remove them entirely, or to repair the damage they have caused. A penile implant is something that you should investigate thoroughly and not enter into lightly. The best thing you can do is to talk to several men who have had one and see how it worked for them and what problems they encountered.

JUNE AND BARBARA: Of course, all these devices may become obsolete with the arrival of Viagra, the new anti-impotency prescription drug approved by the FDA in March 1998. It is the source of a hundred hopes—and hundreds more tasteless jokes. Could you tell us how it works?

VIRGINIA: I'll try to stick to the facts without the jokes. An erection is caused by increased blood flow into certain internal areas of the penis. Viagra enhances the smooth muscle relaxant effects of nitric oxide, a substance that is normally released in response to sexual stimulation. This smooth muscle relaxation allows blood to enter and pool in the penis, leading to an erection. Although Viagra can be taken thirty minutes to four hours before sexual activity, it is generally taken about one hour before, so you do need to plan ahead.

JUNE AND BARBARA: We've never known of a drug that didn't have side effects. What are those associated with Viagra?

VIRGINIA: So far the ones reported include headache, flushing, stomachache, a stuffy nose, diarrhea, and mild and temporary visual changes such as color and light perception change and blurred vision. Most men would consider these side effects a fair trade-off for potency.

JUNE AND BARBARA: Most men *wouldn't* consider death a fair trade-off and almost as soon as Viagra hit the market, there were some deaths reported that seemed to be connected to its use. Could you explain some of the risks associated with taking Viagra and who would be advised not to take it?

VIRGINIA: Men who are using medicines that contain nitrates, such as nitroglycerin, should not take Viagra because the combination of the two drugs may cause a dangerous lowering of blood pressure. As a matter of fact, several medications are known to interact with Viagra, so tell your doctor about any medications—including non-prescription ones—that you're taking to make sure they're not on the interaction list.

JUNE AND BARBARA: Is Viagra covered by most health insurance?

VIRGINIA: As of this writing, it's still being evaluated by insurance providers, but some have already approved its coverage up to a certain number of tablets a week or month. Not to make a sexist remark, but since most of the bodies that decide such things are male bodies, I would be extremely surprised if Viagra wasn't generally approved.

JUNE AND BARBARA: Is there any final advice for men considering taking Viagra?

VIRGINIA: This is both the beginning and the final advice. You should first have a complete medical history and exam to determine the cause of your impotence and make sure it's something that Viagra can help. Also, some men with certain medical conditions such as sickle cell anemia, leukemia, multiple myeloma, or an abnormally shaped penis may not be able to take Viagra. Since this is such a new drug, you can keep informed through newspaper and magazine and Internet reports and questions to your doctor to see if any new problems—or benefits—have been discovered about Viagra.

JUNE AND BARBARA: Now it's the women's turn. Do they also have diabetes-induced sexual problems?

VIRGINIA: Yes, although they're much less common, or at least they're less obvious and less frequently reported. It also may be that women's sexual problems are taken somewhat less seriously by the predominately male medical researchers. On top of that, most doctors may not be as careful about asking their women diabetes patients about sexual problems as they are about asking men. In a commentary in the Vol. 4, no. 1 issue of *Diabetes Spectrum* by L. A. Bernhard, Ph.D., R.N., it was reported that in a survey of physician members of the Diabetes Association of Greater Cleveland, 85 percent of those who responded said they routinely asked diabetic men about sexual difficulties, but only 33 percent routinely asked women.

Another article in that issue of *Diabetes Spectrum*, "The Differential Impact of Diabetes Type on Female Sexuality," described a study that made a surprising finding. Type 1 diabetes was found to have little effect on sexual responsiveness and sexual relationships in women. On the other hand, Type 2 diabetes had "a consistently deleterious effect on both the women's sexual behavior and their sexual relationships." The Type 2 women "viewed themselves as less sexually attractive, were less happy and satisfied with their sexual partner and sex life in general, were less interested in and more likely to avoid sexual activity with their spouse, and were less likely to lubricate adequately and to reach orgasm. . . . Their sexual activity was less varied and, understandably, they developed dyspareunia (discomfort during intercourse) more frequently."

JUNE AND BARBARA: And to think that people always consider Type 1 diabetes the more serious and restrictive and devastating condition! Were any reasons given for this bad news for Type 2 women?

VIRGINIA: The researchers had a number of theories. One was that Type 2 women may experience more of the autonomic neuropathy that prevents adequate lubrication. (The autonomic nerves are the ones that control the heart and blood vessel muscles and the glands.) Another was that Type 2 diabetes may have a more negative effect psychologically and socially because it generally occurs later in a woman's life than does Type 1 and it disrupts long-established relationships. The husband has often been the center of attention in the marriage, and when the focus changes to the wife's diabetes, a certain amount of marital conflict results. On top of that, a Type 2

woman sometimes experiences mood disturbances, especially height-
ened anxiety and depression that may decrease her emotional avail-
ability to her spouse. Still another hypothesis is that because Type 2
diabetes usually happens at middle age or later and is often accompanied by a weight problem, some of the sexual problems may have to
do with a negative self-image, which in turn is caused more by the
problem of being overweight than by diabetes itself.

But before any of you Type 2 women let yourselves get all bent
out of shape over this research and start overanalyzing yourselves and
possibly creating sexual problems that weren't there before, remember that this study was of a total of only 55 women (32 Type 1s and 23
Type 2s) and certain aspects of the findings were in conflict with
findings in other equally reputable studies. But most important,
remember that as Dr. Bernhard said in her commentary on the study,
"each woman is first an individual with her own personal characteris-
tics, and she may not be anything like the group (Type 1 or Type 2) to
which she belongs."

JUNE AND BARBARA: Clearly, if the woman sees that her problem is
a psychological one related to diminished self-esteem, then some
kind of psychological counseling would be in order. But what if it
turns out to be more a physical problem caused by that autonomic
neuropathy you mentioned?

VIRGINIA: Fortunately, this kind of neuropathy is not as common
as peripheral neuropathy—the kind that causes pain and eventual
numbness in the feet and legs—but still it can be quite troublesome
to the diabetic woman, especially when it interferes with her sexual
function or enjoyment. There are creams and jellies, such as the KY
brand, that can aid the lubrication problem. As far as the autonomic neuropathy itself is concerned, the only treatment we can
offer at the moment is the ever-popular, all-time favorite diabetes
panacea: *Get your blood sugars in control!* There are some medications on the horizon (not yet available) that may eventually help
with all kinds of neuropathy. They are called aldose reductase

inhibitors. It's nice to be able to look forward to these, but still nothing beats that well-controlled blood sugar when it comes to combating neuropathy.

JUNE AND BARBARA: This may be a silly question, but can Viagra be of help to women's sexual problems?

VIRGINIA: It's not a silly question. In fact, as soon as Viagra was approved for men, research began on the possible benefits for women. We'll have to wait and see what they come up with. Never underestimate a drug company's interest in doubling the market. But it's only fair that women should have equal consideration. After all, what's sauce for the goose is sauce for the gander. But since this is beginning to verge on a tasteless joke, we'd better move along to the next topic.

FEAR OF INSULIN INJECTION

JUNE AND BARBARA: It's a very important one. Of all the intense emotions that assail people with diabetes, especially Type 2s, one of the greatest is fear of having to take insulin injections someday. Since insulin therapy is the last resort for treating Type 2 diabetes and many Type 2s never have to take insulin, people can have months or years or even a whole lifetime to live with the dread of "going on the needle," as it's often called. They build up a fear that is totally out of proportion to reality. We should know because June experienced that fear for a whole year while she was trying to make it on diet and pills.

Of course, certain individuals actually have a true pathological terror of needles, known as needle phobia among psychologists. What words of comfort do you have for all those people out there living in various states of dread at the thought of taking insulin injections?

VIRGINIA: Many of us who have diabetes and have taken insulin can tell you that it is the least of the issues of having diabetes. As far as we can see, the biggest issue is not about having to take insulin but about not getting to eat brownies. This deserves far more attention and correction than all the emotion and upset surrounding insulin.

Still, I have seen patients who avoid going to the doctor, avoid participating in their own health care, and try to deny their diabetes altogether over the issue of taking a shot of insulin. Granted, taking shots is not everybody's favorite thing to do. If you have been avoiding the doctor out of fear that he or she might say you have to take insulin to get in better control, let me tell you this is one of the biggest nondeals in America today. The insulin syringes are 30- or 31-gauge needles. That's about the diameter of a hair. Ninety-nine percent of the time, with good technique, you literally can't feel them going in and out of your tummy. (Tummies are definitely the best place to give insulin.) So having to use insulin is not an excuse for not being in good control.

One thing we point out to people all the time is that giving an insulin shot, if it hurts at all, hurts a whole lot less than sticking your finger to check your blood sugar. You want to get out there and find the needles that hurt the least and check out the special devices for shooting in the needle. (The effect of these is to give you perfect injection technique.) Try out all the new technology and take advantage of the goodies you find to make insulin injection easier.

I have a lot of patients who say they wish they'd gone on insulin much earlier, because they feel so much better after getting their sugars under control. This improvement in the way they feel overcomes the minor inconvenience of having to give injections twice a day and drives the fear of injecting right out the door.

ADJUSTING TO LOSS OF SPONTANEITY

JUNE AND BARBARA: Over the years, when you talk to people who are discouraged about the things they've lost in life—or *think* they've lost in life because of diabetes—what seems to bother them the most?

VIRGINIA: Although they may tell about it in different ways, it all boils down to just one loss, the only real loss: the loss of spontaneity. That's the ability to do what you want to when you want to do it on the spur of the moment without having to plan ahead and make special arrangements. It can be as simple as spontaneously deciding you'd like to go out to eat in a restaurant and order whatever you feel like at the moment. Or it can be a little more complex, like something I observed a few weeks ago.

I was doing a diabetes program for a hospital in Midland, Texas. We all had a great time, but since it went on all day it was quite strenuous, and I was looking forward to getting a little rest on the one-hour flight to Albuquerque. But the plane had some seats that faced each other, unlike the usual airplane seating where everyone is facing forward and you can catch a little nap if you feel like it. Just my luck, I got one of those seats and a couple plopped down across from me.

This lady was bound and determined that we were going to talk. I mean, she was the original Chatty Cathy. She delighted in telling me that up until thirty minutes ago they had no plans to go to Las Vegas. (The plane was going on to Las Vegas from Albuquerque.) They just got home from work and suddenly decided, "Hey, let's go to Las Vegas for a couple of days."

"So here I am!" she said. "I don't even have any clothes with me. I didn't even have time to put any makeup on." She'd brought her makeup with her and proceeded to put it on right there in the plane. They planned to buy some clothes when they got to Las Vegas. These people had the money, the freedom, and the spontaneity in their life to do that sort of thing. We should all be so lucky to be in the oil business (pronounced "awl bidness" in my part of the country) so we could do just that—if we didn't have diabetes, that is.

Your limitation as a person with diabetes is that you can't just hop in the car, run to the airport, jump on a plane, and go to Las Vegas. No, you'd have to plan your supplies and your injections and your meals. But then, how many of us can jump on planes on the spur of the moment anyway? We have jobs, families, and responsibilities that keep us tied down to a routine. Diabetes can actually be a positive factor to get us organized and stay in touch with reality if we let it.

JUNE AND BARBARA: Yes, it's true, diabetes can organize your life better than any of those books or courses on how to bring order out of your chaotic existence. But if spontaneity is the biggest thing in your life, you can be spontaneous if you plan for it. That sounds like a contradiction in terms, but it really isn't.

People are always telling you to be prepared for any emergency. We're especially conscious of this in California with our earthquakes, but other states have things like tornadoes and hurricanes and floods. You need to be prepared with a kit containing all your diabetes supplies and snacks so you can pick it up and run if disaster hits. We once heard David Marero, Ph.D., a psychologist from Indiana University, speak on being prepared. His theory was, why just be prepared for terrible happenings? The same preparation works for wonderful happenings as well.

Suppose someone says to you, "I want to take you on a horseback ride up into the hills and we'll have a picnic supper and listen to music and watch the sunset." Do you say, "Oh, drat! I can't go. I don't have my insulin (or pills or whatever)"? No, you say, "Terrific. I'll just grab my Spontaneous Happy Event Kit, and we're off."

We know a young diabetic guy who practices what you might call modified spontaneity. He and a buddy pack their bags and his diabetes supplies and they go to the airport and take the next plane that's going somewhere no more than an hour or two away. His diabetes never causes him any problems—at least no more than it would at home.

So you see, spontaneity is possible. But, really, we've found that in the modern world, spontaneity is becoming an overrated commodity. Before June's diabetes diagnosis, we used to travel in Europe by buying a Eurailpass and jumping on a train—any train—and getting off wherever the mood struck us. Then we'd wander around until we found a hotel room. No more. And that's not just because of diabetes. More and more people are traveling, and the hotel you decided to stay in is likely to be *"complet"* as the French say or "fully booked" as the British put it. Ditto for the restaurant you'd like to eat in. If you want to have a really great trip, you need to plan it as carefully as a space launch. That's what we do now, and guess what! It's a lot more fun than winging it. You get weeks and weeks of anticipation as you prowl through guidebooks picking out where you want to visit, corresponding with picturesque hotels in convenient locations, even reserving special restaurants ahead of time. By the time you get there you feel you know the place, and that knowledge sets you free to relax and enjoy yourself.

So if you prefer spontaneity or anticipation or a combination of the two, you can have it in most areas of your life. Diabetes won't stop you. We don't need to envy the "awl bidness" pair—except maybe for their money!

CHAPTER 6

PAYING THE BILL FOR DIABETES:

Dollars and Nonsense

Dealing with the financial aspects of American medical care these days is like walking into a madhouse, and it's beginning to seem like the most violent shock treatments are reserved for people with diabetes. Your first problem is getting health insurance at all, because insurance companies are only willing to insure perfect specimens. It's like the automobile insurance companies wanting to insure only people who've never had an accident and are statistically unlikely to have one.

It's not so bad if you live in a state that has pooled-risk insurance coverage available. Over one-half the states now offer this kind of program. Pooled risk means that any insurance company that wants to do business in a state must contribute to a fund that will issue health insurance to those who would otherwise not be able to obtain it or would only be able to get it for exorbitant rates. They cannot charge more for pooled-risk insurance than 125 to 150 percent of the average health insurance premium in that state.

If you have been rejected for health insurance coverage—either group or individual—you may be eligible for pooled risk, although check on the cost; it varies widely by state. Call your state's

Insurance Commissioner or health department to find out the details for your state.

That's when the craziness begins. An article in the *Los Angeles Times*, "Working Without a Net," described what happened to a self-employed man with the preexisting condition of diabetes. When he quit his previous job to start his own business, the cost of private health insurance for himself and his wife started doubling every three months. When it hit $16,000 a year—just about equal to the amount of his annual income—he had to shut down his business and go to work for a government agency just to get the medical insurance to cover his diabetes.

The article also told of growing numbers of people who are hanging on to jobs they've outgrown or detest, simply to keep their health insurance. It's not only bad for business to have all these unhappy (and therefore less efficient) employees, but it takes all the joy and enthusiasm out of the work life of the employee who is being held a hostage to health insurance.

Even if you like your work and have insurance, your situation still isn't totally sensible and sane. Each year you find your coverage eroding and your deductible and copayment increasing. This is because medical charges are getting out of hand and out of sight. (The *Times* article gave the example of a woman who had a miscarriage and ended up with a $6,000 bill for one night's stay in the hospital. The bill included such charges as $14 for 4 ounces of mouthwash and $17 for a 15-cent sanitary pad.)

And the underlying reason for such exorbitant charges is the essence of nuttiness. Only around one-fourth of hospital patients have private health insurance. Therefore these people pay not only for their own care but for a portion of the care of those who have no coverage and those who have Medicare or Medicaid, whose payments, set by the government, are not adequate by hospital standards. This makes about as much sense as if you went to a restaurant for dinner and when you got your check, you discovered you were being charged to cover meals for three other diners who didn't have enough money to pay the bill.

Insane though the rest of the health-care system may be, Medicare is pure bedlam. June feels that one of the luckiest circumstances of her life is that she worked for a school district that had its own retirement plan, so she never contributed to Social Security. Therefore, she is not eligible for Medicare and remains covered by a private insurance plan, which, although it is not perfect, compared to Medicare it is a thing of beauty (and rationality!) and a joy forever.

The one bright light on the insurance horizon is a significant improvement in Medicare coverage for people with diabetes. In 1997, Congress enacted legislation to cover diabetes education and to provide meters and blood sugar test strips for all diabetics, not just for those who take insulin, as before. This is a true breakthrough for Type 2 people, though we will never fathom why Medicare still won't reimburse for insulin and syringes. It pays for things that show how your blood sugar is doing but not for the only things that may be absolutely essential to keep your blood sugar in control. This is a real puzzler.

We could go on and on spelling out the problems with health care. But better that we do as Barbara used to when we were directors of the SugarFree Centers. If we were going out of town, she always left a list of phone numbers where we could be reached, so that others could "get in touch with us with the solutions to any problems that may have developed in our absence." So we'll ask Virginia to get in touch with you with solutions to the problems associated with the financial aspects of diabetes.

—*June and Barbara*

HEALTH INSURANCE

JUNE AND BARBARA: It would help if you could start with an overview of the kind of health insurance plans that are available, so we can understand what each has to offer.

VIRGINIA: It's important for everyone to understand the different types of insurance, but it's vital for people with diabetes.

Many people have an insurance plan that gives them the option of choosing an HMO (health maintenance organization). For people who have a chronic disease like diabetes, these plans have some advantages and some disadvantages. One advantage is that if you require lots of medications, these programs usually allow you to get them for a nominal copayment (the amount you have to pay out of pocket) of $5 to $10 for each prescription. A disadvantage is that they often operate under a formulary. This means that they have a committee that selects medications for their plan. They make their selections based on effectiveness and price. To achieve cost savings they will select one or two specific drugs from each classification instead of allowing physicians on their plan to prescribe a variety of brand names.

For people with diabetes, this means that you may not get your usual brand of insulin. This is one area in which I see many patients make a mistake. As long as you're receiving human insulin, there's probably no difference between brands and you should get whatever costs less. I've seen patients pay an extra filling fee just to get the particular brand of insulin they've been using. This can turn out to cost more than if they'd just forgotten about their HMO pharmacy service and gone out and bought the insulin retail.

Another way diabetics can cause themselves problems is when it comes to buying syringes. Let's say you prefer a certain brand of syringe, yet the HMO will only give you a lesser quality syringe for your copayment, and you think you're stuck (?!) with that. In fact, syringes are so inexpensive (especially if you shop around and find specials on them, and double especially if you reuse them four or five times) that you can buy them outside your copayment plan.

Where your copayment arrangement comes in handy is for expensive medications like those for high blood pressure. Those can be purchased with great savings on your prescription card.

GENERIC DRUGS

JUNE AND BARBARA: Sometimes this works well when you aren't even on an HMO. Barbara's mother, who has Blue Shield, can get her "maintenance" prescriptions for only $10 each if she buys them through a certain drugstore's mail-order plan. Of course, they prefer to give generics in this case, but if her physician insists, they will provide the exact drug prescribed.

We should mention some of the differences between generic and trade-name drugs. One of the best explanations we've seen is from Mike Voelker, Pharm.D., pharmacist at N.M.C. Homecare in Southern California.

"Generic drugs (drugs not protected by trademark) are in demand today and for many valid reasons. First, insurance companies and other health cost payment systems are encouraging their members to use generic drugs by offering people a lower copayment if they do. Second, the FDA (Food and Drug Administration) is shortening the time period for trade-name drugs to become generic. And, third, over the next three to four years the federal government is phasing in Medicare payments for prescription drugs, and, just as many states do with their Medicaid programs, the federal government will probably demand that generic medications be provided whenever possible.

"For the above reasons it is safe to say that generics are here to stay. But, buyer, beware! Some warnings are in order. Brand-name drugs and their generic forms are not necessarily identical. Switching to a generic without proper precautions may cause serious problems. To understand the possible difficulties, you have to understand what generic drugs are and how they're made.

"A generic drug has exactly the same amount of the active ingredient as the trade-name product. The active ingredient by weight, however, makes up only a fraction of the total weight of the tablet or capsule. For example, a Lanoxin 0.25-mg tablet weighs about 2.5 mg, but the active ingredient, digoxin, makes up only about 10 percent of the total weight of the tablet. The other 90 percent is comprised of what pharmacists call 'excipients'—fillers, binding agents, coloring, etc. It is these extra ingredients that very often determine how much of the active drug is absorbed into the bloodstream and how quickly. In some cases, more drug is absorbed with the generic form, and in other cases less is absorbed. This difference can be very critical, depending on the type of drug.

"With the following classes of drugs you, your doctor, and your pharmacist must be extremely careful when changing to the generic form:

1. Cardiovascular drugs (Lanoxin, Altace, etc.)
2. Hormone and related drugs (Premarin, Synthroid, etc.)
3. Psychotherapeutic drugs (Thorazine, Elavil, etc.)
4. Anticonvulsants (Dilantin, Depakene, etc.)
5. Oral hypoglycemics (Orinase, Diabeta, Micronase, etc.)

"A diabetic, for example, can switch from the trade name Orinase to the generic tolbutamide, but you should always ask your physician first. When the switch is made, you must be very diligent about testing for hyper- or hypoglycemia so that you can determine whether the generic is being absorbed in the same way as the trade-name pill. Then, once you have successfully switched, you have to make sure that you are always provided with that particular brand of generic because the same generics manufactured by different companies also differ in their excipients. This is another complication which means that only those in the know can protect themselves from drug overdose or underdose.

"With classes of drugs *not* on the above list, such as antibiotics and analgesics, it is perfectly OK to switch to a generic brand without any special monitoring.

"The final word on generics, then, is to enjoy the savings they offer, but make sure that you and your physician and your pharmacist work as a team to ensure their safe and efficacious use."

Incidentally, Voelker also told us that pharmacies actually make a greater percentage of profit on generics than on brand names, so if a pharmacist discourages you from purchasing a certain generic, he is doing so for medical reasons and not out of some sordid profit motive.

But let's get off drugs and back to HMOs. What else do we need to know about them?

HMOs

VIRGINIA: Another significant feature is that they use a "gatekeeper" system.

JUNE AND BARBARA: What does that mean? Do they have someone guarding the door who won't let you in unless you can prove you're really sick?

VIRGINIA: It sounds that way, but it's actually a system that requires you to select a primary-care physician (a family doctor or internist). This physician will have to write you a referral before you can go to see a specialist.

JUNE AND BARBARA: Does this mean that you can't just march in and say, "I have diabetes and I want to see an endocrinologist"?

VIRGINIA: That's right. And you can't go directly to an orthopedist when you have a back problem, or to a psychiatrist if you're feeling depressed, and so forth. The reason the HMOs do this is so that the specialists won't be used indiscriminately when a primary-care doctor could have done as good a job. This makes sense. After all, patients aren't always adept at diagnosing their conditions and knowing what kind of specialist—if any—they need. It's also a cost-effective way of providing health care; but if you have a chronic disease like diabetes, it can become a hassle.

JUNE AND BARBARA: It certainly can. We've talked to lots of people with diabetes who belong to HMOs. They know from experience when they need to see an endocrinologist for a diabetes problem, and yet they're slowed down by having to first see the primary-care physician and then wait for him or her to decide that the problem truly is something that requires an endocrinologist's attention, and then wait to get the appointment with the endocrinologist. All the while, the diabetes problem goes untreated. Is there nothing that a diabetic can do to keep this situation from occurring over and over again?

VIRGINIA: Many HMOs in our area allow an endocrinologist to become a primary-care physician for individuals who have an endocrine disease. You should investigate and see if you can work out that kind of arrangement, because it gives you the best of both worlds: the care you need from your endocrinologist or diabetes specialist without the hassles of having to get a referral every time you need to see him or her.

One more thing you need to investigate when choosing an HMO: Look into what they cover. Do they cover your blood glucose meter and strips? The strips are probably the most expensive part of diabetes management.

JUNE AND BARBARA: That certainly is something to look into! We knew of one young woman who was furious because her HMO wouldn't cover her meter and strips. Yet they would cover them for older people on Medicare (those who took insulin), because these people had signed their Medicare benefits over to the HMO and Medicare did cover meters and strips for them. The young woman resented the fact that she, who had a whole lifetime of diabetes ahead of her, was not provided with what was necessary to keep her disease in control, while the older people who had less risk of developing complications were. Obviously, it was more a matter of economics than concern for the well-being of the patient.

Another thing we have noticed about HMOs is that what is covered is often based on what kind of policy you have. Some people say, "I belong to SpendthriftCare HMO so I'll automatically get everything covered." Others lament, "I belong to SkinflintCare and they never cover anything." In many HMOs, some members may have a policy that covers no meters, strips, or prescriptions at all. Others have to pay a portion of the cost. And some lucky devils in the same HMO get virtually everything free of charge. The kind of policy you have, of course, is based on what your employer (or you as an individual subscriber) pays.

You may want to really get serious with your HMO when it comes to specific types of insulin and demand that they provide it even if the insulin brand on formulary doesn't include it, such as the insulin Lispro.

One possible improvement might occur in HMOs if Congress mandates a so-called "patient's bill of rights." As of mid-1998, Congress has just been toying with the idea. The bill of rights would prevent HMOs from putting so many restraints on good care. Keep your fingers crossed.

PRIVATE INSURANCE

VIRGINIA: You could choose a standard indemnity-type insurance plan. This is traditional private insurance. This insurance covers a portion—usually 80 percent—of the costs of hospitalizations and outpatient services such as physicians and prescriptions after you meet a certain deductible. The downside of this kind of policy is that most of the time you must pay cash up front and then get reimbursed, so it can lead to a lot of paperwork.

JUNE AND BARBARA: We once read of a survey that revealed that the thing patients fear most about going to the hospital is not death, but the paperwork they're going to have to handle. We may be cynics, but we suspect that most insurance companies make filing for claims so difficult and keep bouncing back your claims for little niggling details so that you'll become so frustrated and discouraged that you'll just give up and they won't have to pay. Ernest Hemingway once said that if you want to be a writer, you have to be the world's most persistent son-of-a-bitch. The same thing holds true if you want to collect on your insurance.

VIRGINIA: There is an upside, though. With this kind of insurance you have complete choice about the care you get and the physicians and hospitals who give it to you.

JUNE AND BARBARA: But even this kind of policy, which we both have, is starting to "suggest" that you go to certain hospitals and physicians. They have contracted with these providers for a lower rate and the result is "a lower out-of-pocket expense to you." We always try to follow their "suggestion," but even so the "out-of-pocket expense" doesn't seem all that low.

VIRGINIA: That's because of cost shifting, which you touched on in the introduction to this chapter. Since it's referred to so frequently by health professionals and legislators when they talk about the crisis in health care in this country, let me explain in a little more detail what cost shifting is and, more important, why it exists.

Your doctor or pharmacy or other specialist is receiving reimbursement from a variety of sources such as Medicaid, Medicare, HMOs, PPOs (preferred provider organizations), indemnity insurance, and that small category of people who just pay cash. When the doctor receives payment from Medicaid or Medicare, it's been discounted greatly. If his fee for an office visit is $60, he may be getting only $20 from Medicaid for that same visit. The local HMO may be paying him only $35. If you have indemnity insurance you pay the full $60. Of course, you receive $48 back (80 percent of the $60), but only after you've met your deductible. The patient in the waiting room of an HMO will pay maybe $8 or $10 in copayment for the visit.

In the past, indemnity insurance was the preferred way to go. But more and more patients with indemnity plans are discovering that physicians and health-care organizations have to increase their fees to them to compensate for the discounting that's taking place on the other plans—thus you have the term *cost shifting*.

This cost shifting is getting to the point that the indemnity-insured patient is having to pay a higher and higher percentage of the total cost of health care. Those of us who have indemnity plans or pay cash are subsidizing Medicaid and Medicare by more than just our tax dollars. We're subsidizing it every time we go to the doctor or hospital.

Am I saying this cost shifting and subsidizing is good or bad? Neither. I'm just saying that this is how it is. Do I think we need a national health care system? Personally, I don't. When I look at current models of national health care such as the Veterans Administration, military hospitals, Indian Health Service, and the health-care systems in Europe, Scandinavia, and Canada, I don't see any of those systems that I would want to personally participate in. Would I send my child to the VA for health care? I don't think I would. I'm not saying that the VA doesn't have health-care professionals who work hard and care deeply about their patients. What I am saying is that their system is very inefficient and doesn't provide the level of quality care that I would like to see.

JUNE AND BARBARA: But don't you think we need some kind of improvement in our health care system? More and more people—often those with chronic conditions like diabetes—are falling through the cracks and getting no care at all, or else are going bankrupt from paying exorbitant medical costs, losing their homes, and then finally getting public assistance so they can have at least some kind of medical care.

VIRGINIA: I agree that we need something, but first we have to do a much better job with our public health care. It would take so little money, just the cost of one or two heart transplants in every state, to pay for the immunizations that could save a zillion lives. If the money from three or four amputations a year were put into the cost of shoes for people with at-risk feet, it could save the rest of the amputations.

America's health-care priorities need to change. We need to put more money, effort, and concern into preventing disease, into taking care of the basics extremely well—basics like prenatal care, immunizations, and the prevention of chronic diseases.

No, I don't want to see a national health care system like the much-praised one in Canada, where a person must wait two or three years to get gallbladder surgery because it's considered "elective."

JUNE AND BARBARA: It's true that the other systems aren't perfect, and we would want America to do a better job. But can we? Good medical care takes money—more and more every day—and there is less and less of that commodity available in this country.

VIRGINIA: Let me give you an example of how it can be done. At our diabetes program we have a pregnancy program where we work with women who have gestational diabetes and who have diabetic pregnancies. We have a team approach, where we involve the perinatologist (a doctor who specializes in high-risk pregnancies), the endocrinologist, and the nurses and dietitians in the diabetes center. We are able to manage these patients very effectively and monitor them closely and thereby prevent many problems of the diabetic pregnancy. We have normal-weight babies, healthy babies, babies who do not spend time in the Neonatal Intensive Care Unit. Yet with all that we are extremely cost effective. And that's not even considering the long-range cost difference between delivering a healthy baby and an unhealthy one.

JUNE AND BARBARA: But can this be done in a public health care situation?

VIRGINIA: Right now we're working with the Medicaid department in our state, trying to partner with them to help them do a better job of managing their patients in a cost-effective way.

That American Diabetes Association Recognition of Diabetes Education Centers Program I mentioned in Chapter 2 provides a way for third-party payers to know where quality care is being given and to be able to utilize resources more effectively so we get better care at a lower cost.

I think you may see in the future that the third-party payer—whether private insurance or public—will select for you the place where you will go for a certain surgery, the place you will go for your diabetes education, and the places you will go for other specialty kinds of care.

POOLED-RISK AND COBRA INSURANCE

JUNE AND BARBARA: If you have health insurance, but you don't feel that it gives you the kind of coverage you want, is there any alternative or, because you have diabetes, are you pretty much stuck with what you have?

VIRGINIA: First off, you should remember that it's unlikely that you'll ever be totally delighted with your insurance coverage. No one has been since back in the days when some unions were able to negotiate contracts that included 100 percent coverage with no deductible. Those days are gone forever!

I must caution you to investigate very carefully and make certain you can get something else before you give up any insurance coverage. As previously mentioned, many people—especially people with diabetes—will find that they must select or hold on to a job simply for the insurance coverage that it offers.

Even if you're offered a different job that has good insurance and you would prefer to take the new job, you may wind up hanging onto the job you already have because the health insurance with the new company won't cover a "preexisting condition" for the first six months or a year or, in some dismal cases, as long as two years. If you have diabetes, this means your new insurance will be of little value to you during the preexisting condition exclusion period. After all, any health problem that you are likely to have may well be related to diabetes—or the insurance companies will claim that it is.

In 1997, the Kennedy-Kassebaum bill was passed and is supposed to help people with the "portability" of their insurance. If you change insurance plans within a thirty-day period, you can't be denied coverage. Cathy, my business partner in Diabetes Network, and I were able to buy Blue Cross HMO policies for our business with no preexisting condition exclusions (and she has Type 1 diabetes). Pretty good for a couple of old broad diabetics!

JUNE AND BARBARA: We've heard that if a company desperately wants to hire you, you may be able to negotiate a deal with them to pay for your extra coverage during this preexisting condition exclusion period. As Virginia says, though, know what you're getting into before you make any job changes, and, of course, make certain all promises are in writing.

But then, what do you do if the insurance change is not by your choice? What if you get caught in a merger or some other corporate upheaval and get laid off? Are you just left hanging out to dry?

VIRGINIA: No, at least not at first. You can take advantage of the government's COBRA plan. Despite the venomous sound of the name, it can be a lifesaver. COBRA stands for Consolidated Omnibus Budget Reconciliation Act, which, I realize, doesn't explain anything about it. What this plan does is give you the right to keep the insurance from your previous employer for up to eighteen months. The bad news is you have to pay the premium yourself. The good news is that if during this eighteen-month period you have an accident or require surgery with a long recuperation period, the insurance company is obligated to keep covering you until the condition is cleared up.

JUNE AND BARBARA: What if you get laid off and join a new company that has a one-year preexisting condition exclusion? Can you use the COBRA until the preexisting condition period is over?

VIRGINIA: Unfortunately not. The COBRA plan is only for people who have no other health insurance at all. You can't decide to use it just because your new health insurance excludes your diabetes. Supposedly, the Kennedy-Kassebaum bill protects you from that preexisting condition exclusion, but don't forget the thirty-day rule. Pay the COBRA cost to maintain your coverage so when you get your new insurance you will have continuous coverage.

MEDIGAP AND SENIOR PLANS

JUNE AND BARBARA: A lot of people who are on Medicare buy some kind of so-called Medigap insurance to try to plug up the holes in their Medicare. How does this work—or *does* it work?

VIRGINIA: The Feds have fine-tuned their regulations on Medigap plans. They fall into closely defined designations and the company must clearly indicate which plan the customer is getting. Some Medigap plans may cover only the copayment on Medicare-covered benefits. Other Medigap plans may cover expenses not covered under Medicare. Another option is an HMO that will take your Medicare contract for payment. You see these advertised as "senior plans."

The advantage to senior plans is that you get doctor visits and prescriptions for just a small copayment and no paperwork. The disadvantage is that you probably won't get as much choice about your physician. These programs must run very efficiently to make ends meet and therefore they usually offer no-frills care, but that doesn't necessarily mean poor quality. Many times they use nurses for triaging patients in their initial visit, to determine medical priorities, and to make sure they get the correct level of care. Often patients find that they actually prefer getting care from nurses rather than physicians because the nurses do more teaching and spend more time with the patient.

I guess our challenge for the future is how to get Cadillac care for Volkswagen prices. Our health-care system is going to have to become something like a Toyota: efficient, attractive, and moderately priced with excellent quality.

AT MY AGE, WHY SHOULD I BOTHER?

Now that we've come to the end of the questions on Type 2 diabetes, we're left with just one question—the one we've heard more than any other from people who are diagnosed diabetic in their adult years. This question is: "At my age, why should I bother making all these changes?" More specifically, "At my age, why should I start a whole new way of eating? I like the way I've always eaten." Or, "At my age, why should I start exercising? I've never liked exercise. I didn't like it when I was younger and I like it even less now." Or, "At my age, why should I try to lose weight? It's not easy—I should know because I've tried to do it dozens of times, and the weight never stays off anyway." Or, "At my age, why should I stick my fingers and take all those blood sugars? It doesn't feel good and it's expensive." And, finally, "What possible good can doing all these things do me at my age?"

We agree. If you're an oldie, you definitely shouldn't bother. It's a waste of time and it probably won't do you any good at all. Your next question might logically be, at exactly what age do you become an oldie?

That's not an easy one to answer. We've seen oldies who were in their twenties and thirties, and we've seen people in their nineties who were definitely not oldies. June started using the term "oldie" when she herself was in her sixties, and she often used it in reference to people who were much younger than herself. She's always pointing out oldies doing such things as driving about 40 miles per hour in the fast lane of the freeway or unconsciously and inconsiderately blocking supermarket aisles with their shopping carts.

One of her favorite oldie experiences occurred back when we were running the SugarFree Center. June answered the phone one day. It was a woman calling to cancel her appointment to learn how to use a meter. The reason she gave for canceling was, "You see, I'm sixty years old." June, who was sixty-four at the time, mused to herself, "What does being sixty have to do with canceling an appointment? . . . Oh well, I guess she's just an oldie."

When pressed to sum up exactly what an oldie is, June says it's a person who has given up on himself or herself. As we said before, that can happen at any age. But it's true that the older you grow the more temptation there is to fall victim to the oldie syndrome.

If you want to see whether you are developing incipient "oldieism," try taking the following test.

1. Do you use your age as an excuse for getting out of doing things?

2. Do you expect others to do special things for you? That is to say, do you have an "I need to be taken care of" turn of mind?

3. Even if you're financially well off and secure, do you feel poor and hesitate to spend money on *yourself* for things that would make you healthier and happier?

4. Do you use your age as an excuse—even if it's just to yourself—for being unhappy?

5. Do you generally resist trying new things?

6. Do you usually try to avoid responsibility?

7. If you're not retired yet, do you look forward to retirement as a time when you can "just do nothing"? If you *are* retired, do you spend most of your time "just doing nothing"?

8. Do you feel the best part of your life is over?

9. Do you focus on what you can't do rather than on what you can do?

10. Do you feel you're too old and that your mind doesn't work well enough now to try to work new electronic or technological devices—for example, the automatic teller machine at the bank, a computer, a VCR, or, most significantly, a blood sugar meter?

11. Do you often feel sorry for yourself?

12. Do you think more about the past than about the present and future?

13. Do you have a lot of regrets?

14. Do you have more things that you dread than things that you look forward to?

15. Do you often find yourself saying—or even thinking—such phrases as "What's the use?" or "It's just not worth the effort"?

16. Do you feel that you're too old to do most of the things you'd really like to do?

17. Do you primarily think of yourself and *your* needs rather than others and *their* needs?

Count how many yes answers you have. As you may have suspected, this quiz is like one of those "Are you an alcoholic?" quizzes in which even one yes answer is cause for concern. If you answered yes to one or more questions, you either are an oldie or are well on the way to becoming one.

But all is not lost. You don't have to be an oldie. Diabetes may be just the wake-up call you need to push you off the oldie track. We both practice oldie prevention with every fiber of our beings and it must be working at least a little. A few years ago after a talk we gave in Salt Lake City, a woman came up to us and said, "I hope you'll take this in the right way, but from reading your books, I'd think you're a lot younger than you really are." We did take it in the right way—except that she was a little wrong in her assessment. Our real ages are not necessarily the ones that our birth certificates would indicate—and neither is yours. We recently heard a saying attributed to the baseball player/philosopher Satchel Paige: "How old would you be if you didn't know how old you were?" Ponder that one a minute. And then possibly experience a little shudder of horror at the possibility that if you didn't know how old you were, you might be a decade or two older from the way you're conducting your life.

A famous yachtsman once said, "Somewhere in the corner of your heart, you're always twenty-two years old." Now's the time to find that corner and expand it until it occupies your whole heart. Because it still is possible for you to be twenty-two years old in all the ways that really count, and one of the most important of those ways is feeling that many wonderful moments lie ahead for you and starting to take good care of yourself so you can enjoy them to the fullest.

At your age—whatever that age may be—it *is* worth the bother and, more important, *you're* worth the bother.

—*June and Barbara*

A FOND FAREWELL

One of the rules for giving a speech is, "Tell them what you're going to tell them. Tell them. Then tell them what you told them." The same rule holds true for a book. We've done the first two and now we'll end by having Virginia tell you the most important part of what she's already told you. She's doing this in the form of a loving Valentine: "The Fifteen Commandments for Living Well with Diabetes." (She says this means that it's 50 percent more difficult to have diabetes than to be a good Christian or Jew.) We think you should make a copy of this and put it on your refrigerator, bathroom mirror, or some other place where you'll see it frequently.

The Diabetes Gospel According to Virginia Valentine
Virginia's Fifteen Commandments for Living Well with Diabetes

1. Thou shalt find a doctor and diabetes educator who understand that Type 2 diabetes is not a character flaw and who will work with thee to achieve normal range blood sugar goals, and thou shalt honor them.

2. Thou shalt visit thy doctor and diabetes educator every three months for monitoring of thy diabetes with glycohemoglobin and checking for possible complications.

3. Thou shalt work with the dietitian to design a livable yet healthy diet (high fiber, low fat, low protein, low sugar, low salt) that includes goodies now and then so thou won't covet gooey sweets and pig out.

4. Thou shalt have thy blood pressure and cholesterol and triglycerides monitored every three months and follow the diet and medication regimen to get them in the normal range. Also ask thy doctor if thou should be taking a baby aspirin every day to lower thy risk of heart attack.

5. Thou shalt have thy urine checked for microalbuminuria (microscopic levels of protein) every year after five years of diabetes and have any urinary tract or bladder infections treated immediately.

6. Thou shalt see thy ophthalmologist at least annually.

7. Thou shalt care for thy teeth and gums daily and see thy dentist and hygienist every six months.

8. Thou shalt monitor thy blood glucose levels on a regular basis and especially do a test when thou does not want to.

9. Thou shalt check thy feet daily and see a podiatrist every two to three months.

10. Thou shalt wear thy medical ID tag now and forever.

11. Thou shalt not smoke nor take up any tobacco products.

12. Thou shalt get a flu shot every year and thou shalt wear thy seat belt at all times whither thou goest.

13. If thou art woman and thy womb be fertile, thou shalt remember that bad blood sugars beget big bad babies with health problems. Do not beget any babies until thy blood sugars art in perfect control and thy doctor hath blessed any begettin'.

14. Thou shalt do something every day in the way of a healthy and pleasurable activity for thy body, thy mind, and thy spirit.

15. Thou shalt love thyself as a worthwhile person with many wonderful qualities and facets and not flog thyself for having diabetes or for the occasional blooper blood glucose.

AMEN

RECOMMENDED READING AND LISTENING

Note: The following books are available at most major bookstores or from Prana Publications (call 1-800-735-7726 for information). The audiotapes are also available from Prana Publications.

GENERAL BOOKS

Black Health Library Guide to Diabetes by Lester Henry, Jr., M.D., with Kirk A. Johnson (1993) 181 pp.

A guide written expressly for African Americans, one in every ten of whom has diabetes, by the Chief of Endocrinology at Howard University, a man with more than fifty years' experience treating diabetes. His book tells people what they need to know to respect and survive it. A sound, realistic book, very clearly written and with a wonderful philosophy.

Diabetes: A Practical New Guide to Healthy Living by James Anderson, M.D. (1981) 210 pp.

Dr. Anderson, professor of medicine and clinical nutrition at the University of Kentucky, believes diabetics can lead rewarding lives through proper diet and exercise. Features his High-Carbohydrate-Fiber, Low-Fat Nutrition Plan (HCF), which he began developing in 1974. Particularly helpful for overweight non–insulin-dependent diabetics.

Diabetes A to Z by the ADA (rev. ed., 1996) 200 pp.

Tells "What You Need to Know About Diabetes: SIMPLY PUT." Alphabetized for quick reference to over fifty important topics, like food labeling, glycohemoglobin tests, exercise, dental care, blood glucose self-tests, etc.

Diabetes Mellitus: A Practical Handbook by Sue K. Milchovich, R.N., C.D.E., and Barbara Dunn-Long, R.D. (6th ed., 1995) 200 pp.

An easy-to-use, thorough explanation of diabetes and how to control it. Very complete on diet and food choices (includes the entire Exchange Lists); sample meal plans for different calorie levels. Large type. Excellent for beginners.

The Diabetes Sourcebook: Today's Methods and Ways to Give Yourself the Best Care by Diana Guthrie, R.N., Ph.D., and Richard Guthrie, M.D. (3d ed., 1997) 304 pp.

This basic book is distinctive because the Guthries, whom we have known since 1979, have always been at the forefront of diabetes therapy and education. Trust them implicitly to help you in every aspect of daily diabetes care. It's all here from testing equipment to stress management, to food guides, family support, working with your doctor, dental care, sex, and exercise.

The Diabetic Man by Peter A. Lodewick, M.D., June Biermann, and Barbara Toohey (2d ed., 1996) 352 pp.

The guide to health and success in all areas of a man's life:

career, sports, travel, sex, impotence, and relationships. Includes advice, empathy, and support for those with a diabetic man in their lives and for parents of a diabetic son. Dr. Lodewick is an endocrinologist, sportsman, and a well-controlled diabetic.

The Diabetic Woman by Lois Jovanovic, M.D., June Biermann, and Barbara Toohey (rev. ed., 1996) 286 pp.

The only book telling how women can deal with diabetes-related problems at different life stages. Medical advice and realistic coping methods for the complex concerns of today's woman. Includes supplements on Type 1 pregnancy and gestational diabetes. Dr. Jovanovic is an endocrinologist specializing in the problems of diabetic women, a senior scientist at Sansum Medical Research Foundation in Santa Barbara, a diabetic, a wife, a mother, and, as this book shows, a warm, caring person.

The Diabetic's Book: All Your Questions Answered by June Biermann and Barbara Toohey (4th ed., 1998) 275 pp.

A completely revised and expanded edition of the classic book to read when you're first diagnosed diabetic. It's also appropriate for long-term and "born-again" diabetics. An entire section is devoted to people with Type 2 and includes all the new oral hypoglycemic pills. There is also a new section devoted exclusively to the breakthrough low-carbohydrate diet for blood sugar control and weight loss. You'll learn how to select a doctor, how to deal with interpersonal relations and work situations, and how to rebuild your life by coming to terms with the demands of the disease. As Dr. Lois Jovanovic says in her foreword, "June and Barbara will almost make you feel sorry for persons who do not have diabetes!"

The Diabetic's Total Health Book by June Biermann and Barbara Toohey (3d ed., 1992) 302 pp.

The book that proves you can have diabetes yet be the picture of health, leading a vital, productive, happy life. Shows how to focus on health rather than on disease and how to achieve a strong body, tranquil mind, and blithe spirit. Entertaining—and effective!—sections on reducing stress and raising your spirits with travel, laughter, and hugs. Besides the latest in diabetes therapy, there are sections on weight training for all ages, growing your own vegetables with no-work gardening, and thirty-five of June and Barbara's favorite recipes.

How to Get Great Diabetes Care by Irl B. Hirsch, M.D. (1996) 180 pp.
This invaluable manual is a first-of-its-kind. Its title describes perfectly exactly how it will help you. It tells you the best standards of care, explaining what you need to know to demand them of your doctors and nurses and HMO.

The Johns Hopkins Guide to Diabetes by Christopher D. Saudek, M.D., Richard R. Rubin, Ph.D., C.D.E., and Cynthia S. Shump, R.D., C.D.E.
By three professionals from the respected Johns Hopkins University Diabetes Center, this new comprehensive home reference guide is absolutely authoritative and up-to-date. Its unique emphasis is to bring you, the patient, into the picture and to address all of your concerns—medical, financial, and emotional. Everything you need to know for good control, good health, and a good life. (Over thirty illustrations.)

Living with Diabetic Complications by Judy Curtis (1993) 294 pp.
A book for and by people who live with serious diabetic complications. Never dismal, whiny or preachy, it's supportive, informative, and positive. Sound, workable strategies for coping physically and emotionally. Thorough and competent on medical treatment options plus sources of additional specialized help. Judy, diabetic for forty-two years, has experienced vision impairment, kidney and heart disease, neuropathy, and an amputation. She's a perfect role model and an honest and caring writer. Incorporates answers to questionnaires sent to hundreds of people with complications. A one-of-a-kind book.

101 Tips for Staying Healthy with Diabetes by the University of New Mexico Diabetes Care Group (1996) 112 pp.

The inside track on easy-to-follow techniques for preventing and treating complications, in question-and-answer format. Sample subjects include reducing pain of finger sticks, treating and preventing skin infections, and avoiding inappropriate flu and cold medicines.

Reversing Diabetes by Julian Whitaker, M.D. (1987) 389 pp.

Dr. Whitaker, inspired by writings of Nathan Pritikin, has long championed a lifestyle program for diabetics and heart patients based on diet and exercise. At his Wellness Institute in Newport Beach, California, he's treated thousands of patients with his system of a diet high in complex carbohydrates and fiber and an exercise program of four to six days per week. He also advocates vitamin and mineral supplements. Provides the rationale for a high-carbohydrate, low-fat diet and includes a month of menus with over 100 recipes. A complete do-it-by-the-book program.

FOR SPANISH SPEAKERS

La Diabetes y el Cuidado Fácil por Allison Nemic, R.N., B.A., y otros (1992) 154 pp.

This step-by-step guide for controlling diabetes is written for both children and adults. Very easy to read with many illustrations that make for clear understanding.

FOR PEOPLE TAKING INSULIN

Diabetes 101 by Betty Page Brackenridge, M.S., R.D., C.D.E., and Richard O. Dolinar, M.D. (2d ed., 1993) 208 pp.

A diabetes survival guide answering the questions faced by all insulin-takers. Told in true-life stories that are engaging and fun to read. No medical jargon. Includes every aspect of self-care to help you control your diabetes and your life. If the idea of going onto insulin makes your hair stand on end, reading this will make your hair—and all the rest of you—relax.

AUDIOCASSETTES

Getting Started with Humalog by Betty Brackenridge, M.S., R.D., C.D.E., and Kris Swenson, R.N., C.D.E. (1997) 90 min.

Humalog is a new fast-acting insulin every insulin-user should know about. The authors were involved in the clinical trials for FDA approval. This is a step-by-step guide to getting started with Humalog, who's likely to benefit, and how to coordinate with food, and it includes reports of actual patient cases. Special tips such as wherever you inject it, it absorbs at the same rate and eating too much fiber slows down digestion of carbohydrate and may cause a problem. Also covers children, pregnancy, and the pump. Accompanied by useful pamphlet material.

FOR THOSE FOLLOWING THE LOW-CARBOHYDRATE DIET

(See also Type 2 Diabetes, Weight Loss, and Cookbooks: Low Carbohydrate)

Dr. Atkins' New Diet Revolution by Robert C. Atkins, M.D. (1992) 329 pp.

Dr. Atkins believes a disturbed carbohydrate mechanism is responsible for obesity in 95 percent of people. He calls insulin the hormone that makes you fat and blames insulin resistance and hyper-insulinism for the health problems obesity creates, including diabetes. His diet changes the metabolism to correct this. The initial fourteen-day weight loss diet limits you to 20 grams of carbohydrate daily but the maintenance allows 25 to 90 grams. He asks, "On what level of carbohydrate do you feel the best?" Blood sugar control levels in diabetes are up to you, as is the exact diet you end up on. You're the one who personalizes and execute the diet. Includes carbo-counting charts and sixty-six recipes, which are especially good, but he cautions some are high on fat and to be used only as special treats.

Dr. Bernstein's Diabetes Solution: A Complete Guide to Achieving Normal Blood Sugars by Richard Bernstein, M.D. (1997) 400 pp.

During the twenty years we've known him, Dr. Bernstein has come up with one original idea after another, almost always sticking his neck out against prevailing medical opinion. His plan limits carbohydrate to 30 grams daily divided 6–12–12 for the three meals. He insists on a blood sugar goal of 85–90, the same as nondiabetics. Along with clear, detailed instructions on how to handle virtually every aspect of caring for Types 1 and 2 diabetes, he reveals several surprise benefits such as increased alertness, relief from chronic tiredness, improved short-term memory, a new sense of well-being, and wonderful reassurance that diabetics are not doomed to disabling complications and premature death.

Protein Power by Michael Eades, M.D., and Mary Dan Eades, M.D. (1998) 338 pp.

This eye-opening, scientifically convincing low-carbohydrate book describes how this dietary approach manages obesity, Type 2 diabetes, heart disease, high blood pressure, and elevated cholesterol. A wonderfully complete manual explaining that the diet works by restricting carbohydrate to reduce the body's insulin production. Detailed instructions and formulas for designing your own meals with adequate protein, carbohydrate, fiber, and "good" fats. Includes meal plans, snack foods, a mini-cookbook, and vitamin and mineral supplements. A reliable guide to all you need to know and do for successful weight and blood sugar control for Type 2s, with much useful information for Type 1s.

The Type II Diabetes Diet Book by Calvin Ezrin, M.D., and Robert E. Kowalski (2d ed., 1997) 304 pp.

Dr. Ezrin, an eminent endocrinologist, is one of the pioneers in using a low-carbohydrate diet for weight loss. His new book is directed toward Type 2s who are at least 20 percent overweight. His research and clinical experience have taught him that such people suffer from an identifiable hormonal disorder called "hyperinsulinism."

His Insulin Control Diet is a way to reverse hyperinsulinism so that the body can switch gears and start to burn excess fat as fuel. The diet ensures weight loss of up to 3 pounds per week for women and 4 pounds for men "without much hunger at all." Only 40 grams of carbohydrate are allowed daily but 50–75 grams of protein are included and fat is restricted. In combination with the diet is a non-intimidating exercise plan and relaxation techniques. Includes meal plans, food charts and recipes, plus switching to a stabilization phase.

AUDIOCASSETTES

The Bernstein Plan: Types 1 & 2 by Richard K. Bernstein, M.D. (1995)
     Type 1: Dr. Bernstein clearly explains his good control regimen: the low-carbohydrate diet, muscle-building through anaerobic exercise, multiple blood sugar tests, multiple small doses of insulin, how to prevent hypoglycemia, sick days, and understanding gastroparesis. Order this if you are a Type 2 on insulin. (2 tapes, 90 min. each.)
     Type 2: Incorporates the same principles as Type 1. If medication is needed, metformin is used. (If you take insulin, use the Type 1 tapes.) Discusses how to break the obesity cycle by cutting carbohydrates to reduce hunger, normalize blood sugar, and lose weight and how to reduce insulin resistance by building lean body mass (2 tapes, 90 min. each.)

The Low Carbohydrate Diet for Type 2 Diabetes by Linda Sherman, R.D., Psy.D. (1996) 45 min.
     A basic introduction to a non-extreme, low-carbohydrate diet for weight loss, blood sugar control, and other health benefits. Dietitian Linda Sherman, who works with Dr. Judith Reichman of Cedars Sinai Medical Center in Los Angeles, has taught this eating plan for fifteen years and uses it herself. Linda clearly explains what to eat, when, and why in the three stages of the diet: 1) weight loss, 2) stabilization, and 3) maintenance. This plan allows for total individualization. A typical day of meals clarifies the concept and gives you a true taste of this eating style. A simple written guide accompanies the tape.

INSULIN PUMPS

The Insulin Pump Therapy Book edited by Linda Fredrickson, M.A., R.N., C.D.E. (1995) 160 pp.

If you're on an insulin pump or thinking about using one, this book of "Insights from the Experts" is vital. From the Professional Education Department of MiniMed Technologies, it's a phenomenal reference loaded with the most timely and sophisticated information. Eighteen leading experts with well-deserved worldwide reputations tell you what they know about setting insulin dosages, preventing hypoglycemia, exercise and insulin adjustment, carbohydrate counting, and pregnancy.

Pumping Insulin by John Walsh, P.A., C.D.E., and Ruth Roberts, M.S. (2d ed., 1994) 156 pp.

Many people in the Diabetes Control and Complications Trial that proved the benefits of tight control used a pump instead of syringes for their insulin. Written by a ten-year veteran pump-user, this revised edition gives you all the information you need for deciding whether or not to go onto a pump and the tools you need for its successful use.

TYPE 2 DIABETES
(See also For Those Following the Low-Carbohydrate Diet and Weight Loss)

Managing Type II Diabetes by Arlene Monk, R.D., C.D.E., et al (rev. ed., 1996) 184 pp.

A mine of the latest therapies and strategies for living with Type 2 diabetes. Understandable and encouraging. Explains "routine maintenance" and makes you a genuine partner with the professionals who help you. Includes such innovative illustrations as an "Activity Pyramid" for the exercise aspect of self-care, an excellent survey of all medications, and especially helpful blood glucose testing tips. Reflects the latest advances from the staff of the International Diabetes Center in Minneapolis.

WEIGHT LOSS
(See also For Those Following the Low-Carbohydrate Diet and Type 2 Diabetes)

The Fit or Fat Woman by Covert Bailey and Lea Bishop (1989) 151 pp.

Coauthored with biologist and nutrition counselor Lea Bishop, this book applies Covert Bailey's successful weight loss strategy to women, acknowledging that "women have more trouble with fat than men." The focus of this program is to lower your body's percentage of fat and increase its percentage of muscle. This requires about sixteen months of daily aerobics and a low-fat, low-sugar diet. Special sections on depression, PMS, anorexia, and bulimia. The science is right up-to-date and the fitness advice works and feels good.

The New Fit or Fat? by Covert Bailey (rev. ed., 1991) 167 pp.

The essential message of this well-researched, breakthrough book is that overweight people should concentrate on losing body fat, not pounds. Bailey says that fat people often eat less than skinny people and the only way they can lose body fat is through exercise that changes their metabolism to burn more fat. "The ultimate cure for obesity is exercise."

Weight Management for Type II Diabetes by Jackie Labat, M.S., R.D., and Annette Maggi, M.S., R.D. (1997) 176 pp.

Combines nutrition and exercise in a weight control book specifically for Type 2 diabetics. Covers setting reasonable exercise goals, keeping pace with an exercise regimen, learning to deal with lapses, developing lifestyle habits that last, managing stress, teaming up with others for support, and handling special occasions. Includes an "enlightened shopping tour" and a low-fat cooking lesson. Emphasizes taking action yourself with quizzes and worksheets to create your own weight management success story.

DIABETES AND YOUR EMOTIONS

Diabetes: Caring for Your Emotions as Well as Your Health by Jerry Edelwich, M.S.W., and Archie Brodsky (1986) 276 pp.

This is about the *experience* of diabetes and the "inner drama" of people who suffer from it. Covers a great range of emotional reactions and dilemmas engendered by living with diabetes. Distinguishes between the unique problems of those with Type 1 and Type 2 diabetes as well as their many common grounds. Excellent on doctors and nurses and family relationships and support groups.

Psyching Out Diabetes: A Positive Guide to Your Negative Emotions by Richard R. Rubin, Ph.D., C.D.E., June Biermann, and Barbara Toohey (2d ed., 1997) 384 pp.

We've come to believe that diabetes control is 90 percent in your head! This exciting book helps you straighten out your head and get rid of the fear, denial, depression, grief, frustration, embarrassment, and guilt that block good diabetes control and a good life. If you're used to seeing diabetes as an enemy, something that complicates your already complex life, this book will show you how to improve your perspective, giving you seven specific frames that will enable you to look at your diabetic challenges in a completely different way. Dr. Rubin, a certified mental health counselor on the faculty of the Johns Hopkins Medical School and in private practice in Baltimore, Maryland, has been counseling diabetic patients for over twenty years. Because he has a diabetic son and a diabetic sister, he has lived with diabetes and knows whereof he speaks—and he speaks clearly, directly, and without any psychological mumbo jumbo.

Reflections on Diabetes by the ADA (1996) 104 pp.

You may see your own reflection in this collection of personal essays written by people with diabetes who want to share with others their personal experiences in diabetes, relating high moments and low moments and giving their insights and philosophies of overcoming and enduring. All were published in the *Diabetes Forecast* magazine. Learn from others and gain more equilibrium yourself. Perfect for use with support groups and diabetes classes.

AUDIOCASSETTES

Good Times Therapy by June Biermann and Barbara Toohey (1994) 60 min.

Do you feel that life after diabetes is a drag and a downer? Then you need a shot of our "Good Times Therapy." This is not some far-out California idea but is based on the latest research by psychologists who've discovered that pleasure and the optimism it creates improve your immune system and extend your life. Here, before a live audience, we help you turn off negative forces and turn on joy. We even show how diabetes can actually become the key to realizing your life's dreams.

Psyching Out Diabetes by Richard R. Rubin, Ph.D., C.D.E. (1994) 90 min.

No one speaks more informatively or entertainingly about "Diabetes Overwhelmus"—the emotional battle fatigue of all diabetics—than master storyteller Dr. Richard Rubin, our collaborator on *Psyching Out Diabetes*. Dr. Rubin makes you feel mentally refreshed and more positive about diabetes than you ever thought possible.

SPORTS AND EXERCISE

The Diabetes Sports and Exercise Book by Claudia Graham, C.D.E., M.P.H., Ph.D., June Biermann, and Barbara Toohey (1995) 240 pp.

This is an updated version of our popular 1977 book, which was based on the sports experiences of 168 diabetic exercise enthusiasts. They were the only people who could give help and counsel at that time, since medical science did not recognize the importance of exercise for diabetes control and well-being. This 1995 edition contains the new scientific and technical information about exercising with diabetes and teaches how to attain the marvelous therapeutic effect of exercise. Claudia Graham has a Ph.D. in Exercise Science and is a diabetic who enthusiastically practices sports. She tells you exactly how to use sports to the best advantage and how to avoid any possible negative outcomes. Special chapters for children, those with complications, and older diabetics.

Diabetes: Your Complete Exercise Guide by Neil F. Gordon, M.D., Ph.D., M.P.H. (1993) 137 pp.

Exercise plus diet are the prime therapies for diabetes. There are scores of food books, but fewer than a half dozen exercise books for people with diabetes. What a crazy imbalance! That's why we love this authoritative guide from the famous Cooper Aerobics Center in Dallas. Reveals the real physical payoffs from exercise and how to begin a program and stick with it. Comprehensive, state-of-the-art advice for both Type 1s and Type 2s.

The Fitness Book by the ADA (1995) 149 pp.

Fitness is a necessary goal of all people with diabetes. Claudia Graham, who wrote the chapter on special needs, defines fitness as "the capacity to meet successfully the present and potential challenges of life." A fitness program has three main elements: stretching, aerobic activity, and muscle strengthening. *The Fitness Book* coaches you into shape without undue sweat or tears.

COOKBOOKS: MAINSTREAM AND LOW FAT

The Art of Cooking for the Diabetic by Mary Abbott Hess, M.S., R.D., F.A.D.A. (3d ed., 1997) 560 pp.

This new edition of the best-selling classic has the latest ADA nutritional guidelines and 375 healthful and flavorsome recipes (low cal, low fat, high fiber). It's the *Joy of Cooking* for the diabetic cuisine with a half million copies sold (like having a master chef and a registered dietitian in your kitchen).

Diabetic Cookies by Mary Jane Finsand (1994) 160 pp.

This is a book for true Cookie Monsters. Talk about variety—207 recipes: 74 drop cookies, 75 bar cookies, 33 shaped cookies, and 25 refrigerator cookies. Mainly sweetened with granulated sugar substitute and/or fructose. Easy, complete directions and nutritional analysis. Most cookies have only 4 grams of carbohydrate.

The Diabetic Sweet Tooth Cookbook by Mary Jane Finsand (1993)
A delectable array of cakes, frostings, cookies, candy, crepes, pies, ices and sherbets, drinks, sweet breads, and puddings. Includes personal tips and tricks as well as invaluable conversion guides and recommended flavorings, extracts, herbs, and spices.

Free and EQUAL Cookbook by Carole Kruppa (2d ed., 1994) 132 pp.

Update of the highly popular cookbook featuring dishes made with Equal (NutraSweet). The author grew up and learned her cooking in France, and it shows in the good taste of these 160 low-calorie and sugar-free recipes. Includes breakfast treats, appetizers, soups, salads, entrees, desserts, beverage, jams, and jellies. Calorie counts and exchanges for all recipes.

The Joy of Snacks by Nancy Cooper, R.D. (1991) 285 pp.

If you're a Type 2, snacking six to ten times a day is actually better for you than three square meals. Type 1s need snacks to prevent or treat low blood sugar episodes. Here's the perfect book for both types by an acclaimed dietitian. Lots of muffin and cookie recipes and a large selection of popcorn treats and special snacks for kids. Two hundred great recipes with exchanges.

Magic Menus for People with Diabetes by the ADA (1996) 256 pp.

This book is similar to their previous *Month of Meals* series, only better since it's all in one compact volume. Gives 50 different breakfasts, 50 lunches, 75 dinners, and 30 snacks. You can flip back and forth to any combination of breakfast, lunch, and dinner choices and the total calories will equal 1,500 (levels can be adjusted up or down to suit individual needs). Forget figuring fats, calories, and exchanges; it's all done for you automatically—it's truly like magic.

Quick and Delicious Diabetic Desserts by Mary Jane Finsand (1992) 190 pp.

Scores of recipes for pies and puddings, cakes and cookies, ice cream, and tortes. No meal is complete without one of these luscious treats. Exchanges given.

Vegetarian Cooking for People with Diabetes by Patricia LeShane (rev. ed., 1994) 143 pp.

Over 100 true vegan recipes without dairy products or eggs, emphasizing low-fat cooking. Soy milk, nuts, grains, and legumes are used for protein. Sweeteners are small amounts of blackstrap molasses or honey. Sample dishes: grainburgers, millet with tofu and mush-rooms, soybean mushroom pilaff, apple-oat drop cookies, and rice pudding. The recipes are easy-to-prepare with exchanges and fat per-centages given for each.

COOKBOOKS: LOW-CARBOHYDRATE DIET

Carbohydrate Counting Cookbook by Tami Ross, R.D., C.D.E., and Patti Geil, R.D., C.D.E.

Two highly experienced dietitians of the University of Kentucky who specialize in diabetes have seen the light and focus their book on carbohydrate counting as the key to good control (Amen!). A step-by-step introduction to carbohydrate counting plus 125 appropriate recipes containing from 0–61 grams of carbohydrate per serving. Most recipes are over 15 grams of carbohydrate and are also low fat.

Dr. Atkins' New Diet Cookbook by Robert C. Atkins, M.D., and Fran Gare, M.S. (1994) 248 pp.

Over 200 of the most asked for recipes at the Atkins Center for Complementary Medicine in New York City. They appear non-dietetic because they are not fat restricted—the fat content is not even included—but they are carbohydrate restricted. There are seven kinds of hamburgers and such other high-protein recipes as roast turkey with almond stuffing and tuna meat loaf. Desserts include cheesecake, brownies, chocolate sponge layer cake, and coconut cream pie.

Dr. Atkins' Quick & Easy New Diet Cookbook by Robert C. Atkins, M.D., and Veronica Atkins (1997) 213 pp.

In this low-carbohydrate cookbook, Dr. Atkins' Russian-born wife brings an international flare to the diet, including pleasurable desserts like Shortcake Veronique with a Kiss of Rum. One hundred sixty recipes in all, with carbohydrate analysis. Tips for modifying other recipes to low-carbohydrate dining. Spiral bound.

The Low-Carb Cookbook by Fran McCullough (1998) 384 pp.

Fran McCullough takes the foods you *can* eat and makes them into something you *want* to eat, bringing her years of experience as a cookbook writer and editor to this ideal low-carb guide. Over 250 recipes with tips and cooking skills to inspire some of your own ideas. Includes sweeteners and how to use them most effectively, what to drink, how to cope with entertaining and holidays, sources of low-carb products, and how to deal with plateaus.

FOOD GUIDES AND NUTRITIONAL ANALYSIS

The Carbohydrate Addict's Gram Counter by Richard F. Heller, Ph.D., and Rachael F. Heller, Ph.D. (1993) 90 pp.

The authors are both professors at Mt. Sinai School of Medicine, N.Y. This comprehensive guide gives the calories, fat, and carbohydrate counts for 2,700 foods, including many brand names. It also gives an analysis of menu items from fourteen fast-food chains. It indicates items that are low-fat and heart healthy. Accurate information was supplied by the U.S. Department of Agriculture, U.S. Centers for Disease Control, and other authoritative sources. Easy to use and carry in your pocket or purse as it's only 6" x 4".

Carbohydrate, Calories and Fat in Your Food by Art Ulene, M.D. (1995) 682 pp.

No matter what you count, be it calories, carbohydrates, or fats, this is your master reference guide—30,000 entries in a brand-new edition. Easy to use. Includes brand-name and specialty foods, low-fat foods, and snacks. Over 40 different kinds of peanut butter alone!

Convenience Food Facts by Arlene Monk, R.D. (rev. ed., 1997) 456 pp.

A humdinger reference book. Tells all you need to know about everything in your grocery cart—calories, carbohydrate, fat, cholesterol, sodium, and exchanges. Over 3,000 popular brand-name products plus diabetically oriented ones like Estee.

Exchanges for All Occasions: Your Guide to Choosing Healthy Food Anytime, Anywhere by Marion Franz, M.S., R.D., C.D.E. (4th ed., 1997) 384 pp.

Never has so much sound, authoritative guidance for diabetes eating been packed into one book. The latest nutritional facts and recommendations, including carbohydrate counting. Covers every eating situation and most cuisines (Jewish, Southwestern, vegetarian, etc.). Includes sample menus and twenty-nine recipes.

Fast Food Facts by Marion Franz, R.D. (4th ed., 1994) 182 pp.

A pocket-size guide (4" x 6") for making the right food choices at fast-food restaurants. Complete nutritional information on over 1,500 menu offerings from the fifteen largest fast-food chains. Symbols designate items high in salt, fat, or sugar.

Fat & Fiber in Your Food by Art Ulene, M.D. (1995) 737 pp.

The only comprehensive guide to the magic dietary ingredient, fiber, and the suspect one, fat. You need 20–35 grams of fiber daily to smooth out blood sugars and lower weight and cholesterol. With this book you can get off the fat kick and on the fiber advantage. Thirty thousand entries, including brand-name, generic, prepared, specialty, and fast foods.

The Restaurant Companion by Hope S. Warshaw, R.D. (2d ed., 1995) 360 pp.

Focuses on restaurant dining, showing how to make healthy choices for seven kinds of ethnic cuisines (Mexican, Chinese, Italian, Thai, etc.), as well as vegetarian, American, and fast-food restaurants. Advice for handling salad bars, pizza places, brunches, and airline meals.

AUDIOCASSETTES

Carbohydrate Counting by Betty Brackenridge, M.S., R.D., C.D.E. (1995) 60 min.

Describes this increasingly popular system of meal planning that gives you more mealtime freedom and better control. Reveals how, in spite of its simplicity, just counting grams of carbohydrates (CHO) can help you zero in on the good diabetes control that may have been eluding you. The rationale is that CHO foods (sugars and starches) have a much greater effect on blood sugar than protein and fat. Counting CHO will show those of you who are "playing pancreas" with numerous insulin injections how to adjust your doses to the CHO you eat. The system also works for Type 2s by helping them match their food to their bodies' ability to produce insulin. Covers food label-reading, measuring portions, gram counting books, and adapting the Exchange System to Carbohydrate Counting.

New Nutritional Guidelines by Betty Brackenridge, M.S., R.D., C.D.E. (1995) 60 min.

If you're confused by the big changes in diet for diabetics announced in the 1994 ADA Guidelines, here's help. Dietitian Betty Brackenridge answers the most commonly asked questions such as, "What do you mean there's no more diabetic diet?" "What do you mean I can eat sugar?" "What do you mean I don't need to be my 'ideal weight'?" The 1994 guidelines are far more user-friendly than the old and will bring back dining pleasures you thought were gone forever.

INDEX

C

Calcium channel blockers, 18
Callus and getting blood, 38
Calories, 112-13
Carbohydrates, 108-109
  controlling, 127-128
  counting, 113, 121-23
  foods, 111
  needs and capacities, 125
  slow, 109
Care managers, 28
Cats, eating like, 119-120
CDC (Centers for Disease Control), U.S., 5
Charges, underlying reason for exorbitant, 162
Check strips, 40
Cheese, 102
Cheesecake, 115
Chemstrips bg, 33
Children, goals for, 24
Cholesterol, 17-18
COBRA (Consolidated Omnibus Budget Reconciliation Act), 176
  insurance, 173-174
Coma, diabetic, 4-5
Conscious relaxation exercise, 147-150
Consumer Reports, 64
COPD (chronic obstructive pulmonary disease), 46
Cost shifting, 170
Counters, fat gram, 101
Counting
  calories, 113
  carbohydrate, 121-123
  carbohydrates, 113
Crystal Lite's citrus blend flavor, 112

D

DCCT (Diabetes Control and Complications Trial), 22-23

Denial, 132-136
  hard-core, 136
  parable of, 133
  in reference to diabetes, 134
Deprivation mode, 107-108
Diabeta pills, 95
Diabetes
  defined, 1
  definitions of, 3-10
  diagnosis, 135
  difference between two types, 2
  gestational, 172
  having a positive impact on lives, 140
  and hypertension, 16-19
  keeping knowledge of disease private, 142-143
  lighten up, 141-142
  people who get, 14-16
  regular screening of population for, 5
  Type 2, 1-19
  undiagnosed, 6
  ways and means of controlling, 21-64
Diabetes Center, 41
Diabetes education
  and insurance companies, 43
  Medicare pays for, 41-42
Diabetes Education Centers Program, 172
Diabetes educators, 41
Diabetes Network, 97
Diabetic
  coma, 4-5
  feet, 81
  foods, 113-114
  noncompliant, 94
  shenanigans, 22
Diabetologists, 25-26
Dietary
  confusion, 92
  supplements, 118
Dietetic foods, 113-114